Entries/Entrées
LEAVE TO ENTER FOR SIX MONTHS
EMPLOYMENT PROHIBITED
(79)
15 AUG. 1995
JUL 27 1996

Journey

Journey

An Adventure of Love and Healing

Timothy Todd Tattersall

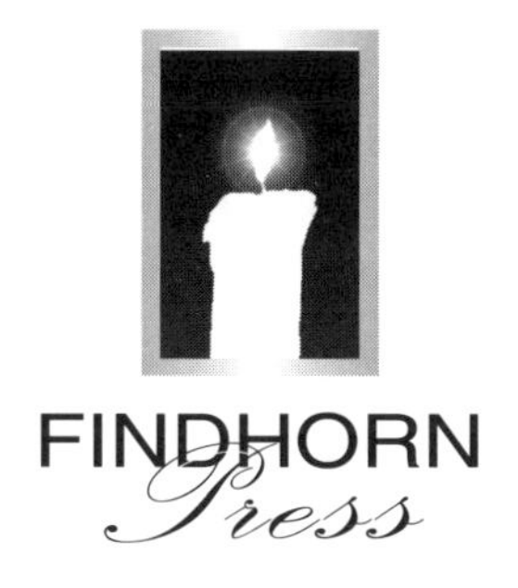

First published 1997
Second impression 1997
ISBN 1 899171 56 8

British Library Cataloguing-in-Publication Data.
A catalogue record for this book is available from
the British Library.

Set in Italia Book by Findhorn Press
Cover design by David Gregson
Cover illustration from *The Book of Kells Colouring Book*,
by kind permission of Bookmark, Cork, Ireland.

Printed and bound by Interprint Ltd. Malta.

Published by
Findhorn Press
The Park, Findhorn,
Forres IV36 0TZ
Scotland
tel +44(0)1309 690582/fax 690036
e-mail thierry@findhorn.org
http://www.gaia.org/findhornpress/
or http://www.mcn.org/findhorn/press/

Contents

We would like to make it clear that when 'Findhorn' is mentioned in this book, in most cases it refers to the Findhorn Foundation and the community that has grown up around it, and not to the nearby village of Findhorn, which has its own history and traditions.

For Grete and Daniel

Acknowledgements

Journey represents for me a labor of love. It would have been impossible to have written it without the guidance and inspiration of several friends. I thank Carolyn, David, Frank, Frankie and my mom. But most especially, my gratitude goes to Carin, who contributed many hours of her time. Not only did she share her writer's expertise, but she also helped me look deeper within my own soul. My warmest thanks to all of you.

— Timothy Todd Tattersall

10

Angels

I stepped off the plane and down onto the tarmac. The warm summer sun shone brightly and I felt every ray fall upon my being on that beautiful and clear August day. At the bottom of the steps I paused to take in the view. Immediately I sensed this would be no ordinary holiday. I was still not quite sure why I had come, but the reality was that I was in Inverness, Scotland.

My immediate surroundings were captivating. The hilly and often mountainous countryside provided a graceful yet dramatic backdrop that was grassy and rocky at the same time. The North Sea lay peacefully just behind me — I could easily follow the coastline where the cobalt blue water contrasted so sharply with the land. A few moments before, as we prepared to land, I had peered through the window. Miles of meandering waist-high stone walls, built perhaps to separate the sheep from the cattle, formed intricate patterns as they darted up and over the mountains. I wondered how long ago they had been created with such painstaking care, and whether the builders would have changed anything if they could have seen their work from my perspective. Probably not. Even on the ground I found low walls providing a sense of security as they surrounded each home. The Scottish flowers of summer stood in full bloom. They seemed so carefree as they swayed gently back and forth in the wind. It is in such a setting that I found Findhorn.

Malin, a friend of mine, had spent a week at the Findhorn Foundation several months before. I didn't understand at the time why she had gone, much less how she had heard about this place in the northern reaches of Scotland. It seemed so distant to me. Yet I remember her enthusiasm when she returned home. She told of the wonderful people she had met, and what an open and loving environment Findhorn had provided for her. Little by little, I learned that the Findhorn Foundation is an international spiritual community that has been in existence in Scotland since 1962. Nearly 350 people live, study and work together year round in this place that was originally known for its work with plants and communication with nature. It has always had strong spiritual foundations as well and over the years has evolved into a holistic educational center. The programs offered to people are based on the same premise that made the original work with nature so successful. My friend assured me that there is a definite and positive energy that emanates physically and spiritually from there.

Findhorn offers a variety of courses for people from outside the community to participate in, but the first course must always be what they call Experience Week One. Malin told me that if I were ever to go there, enrolling in their one-week course would enable me to begin to understand the power of Findhorn. There are many other courses that are available to choose from after one has done the first Experience Week. The variety of programs ranges from aromatherapy and massage to relationships to leadership skills. They even travel with groups to Russia, India and Africa. Findhorn simply offers an open environment that encourages love, truth and honesty for people to step briefly out of *normal* society. It is therefore possible to pause and analyze one's personal growth from the soul's perspective.

As summer neared and I was in conversation one day with Malin, she asked what I had planned for my holidays. I confessed I didn't yet know.

"Why don't you go to Findhorn in Scotland and do an Experience Week like I did?" she suggested.

Although I didn't comprehend it at the time, looking back

I know that is when the first chapter of my life came to a close, and the next opened so dramatically. Without hesitation, without question, without a concrete reason for why I had to go — I just knew that I must — I called the Findhorn Foundation and enrolled in an Experience Week in August. The direction of my life changed from one moment to the next when I made that decision to go. I hadn't the least idea of what to expect; I simply knew the feeling inside was right. Never would I have guessed the events that were about to unfold before me on my journey, my odyssey.

Three weeks before I departed, I had my astrological chart drawn up for me. It had not been done for a few years so I decided it was time. The purpose is not to predict the future — rather, when my chart is read in this manner, it gives me clarity and insight into my life at the current moment. My astrologer also had a new computer program that enabled him to place my personal birth chart directly onto a world map. It is called astrocartography.

"Wow," I said as he produced my map onto his screen. "It's beautiful."

He smiled as he recognized that this map was new to me.

"It is," he responded, "because of the wide rainbow of colors."

All the continents and countries were vividly detailed, and the intersecting lines all had their own unique palette. Maps have always fascinated me, but this one was special.

"Look for the intersections of the fixed latitudinal and the unregulated longitudinal lines," he explained. "Each line has a particular planetary influence. They are all clearly labeled."

As a result, I saw geographically on a world map where my strong energy areas lie. These energy centers range from places that would simply be good to visit, to places where it would be very advantageous for me to live.

"Follow your sun line as it comes up through Brazil and crosses the Atlantic," he guided me as his finger pointed at the screen. "It then jets straight through Ireland and Scotland, and continues through Norway. Those specific countries would be powerful places for you to visit."

"That's interesting," I said, "because I'm going to Scotland in a few weeks."

He laughed. "You'll be very relaxed and inspired there — good choice!"

Never having seen this type of map before, I asked him to print mine for me to keep.

Though born in Florida, I had not one longitudinal or latitudinal line that approached within a thousand miles of there. The two most influential intersections of these lines, for my birth-chart, crossed each other precisely in only one place on the globe, and that is where I live — Italy.

"It's amazing," he said, "that you are an American who lives in Italy. You weren't born here, but according to the map, it is by far the best place for you to reside — a definite alignment of your own fate and destiny."

The second most influential place for me to be was Norway.

"Have you ever been to Norway?" he asked.

"No."

"Have you ever met any Norwegians?"

"No." I thought it strange I had never met a Norwegian.

"If you ever go to Norway, or even if you ever meet a Norwegian outside of Norway, you may possibly feel a strong bond with them."

Never having considered Norway in my life, suddenly this man had piqued my curiosity. Why Norway? Why Norwegians?

The Florence to London flight was easy. I stayed with my good friend David. He had known of Findhorn for years, but had not yet taken the time to go there. He was very excited for me, and his enthusiasm gave me strength. We planned to meet and travel together when I was done in Scotland. An early Saturday morning flight out of Heathrow airport was to take me on the one daily non-stop to Inverness. As it happened, I awoke late, and knew I wasn't off to a promising start. The Underground in London, the subway system that connects the whole of the city, frequently takes longer than usual during non-peak hours. At precisely the time my flight was to leave, I arrived at the wrong terminal at Heathrow. Frantically I asked the ticket agent to call the other terminal and tell them I was on my way because I could not miss the flight.

"You're too late," she confirmed smugly without even a glance at the computer. "We don't hold flights for late passengers, and there is no way you'll make it because the correct terminal is 20 minutes away."

Stunned at her negativity, I countered, "There is no way? Yes, there *is* a way."

I turned around quickly and raced across the marbled concourse. Sweating and angry at myself, I couldn't believe it possible that I would miss the one daily flight to Inverness — and therefore my first day at Findhorn. *I am on that airplane, I am on that airplane,* flashed through my mind repeatedly in those blind 20 minutes. Finally at the gate, with beads of sweat streaming down my face and body, I was overwhelmed to see that the passengers were only just then beginning to board my flight. It was a full 25 minutes past departure time. As I stumbled on board, the captain's voice blared through the intercom to apologize for the delay: the hot-water burner in the galley had broken and had finally been repaired — as a result, we could have our tea en route. I laughed to myself as I realized I would be able to make it to Findhorn on time because of such a minor repair — and the British penchant for tea. With a smile on my face I closed my eyes. I had believed there must be a way, and the path had been made open for me.

Later in my evolving journey, I realized that this was the beginning of my conscious awareness that I create my own dreams and realities. I am totally responsible for what happens to me. Ten years before I moved to Italy, somehow I knew I would live in Europe one day. Although not exactly sure where, I simply knew I would.

When my world map was made, highlighting the powers of specific countries, I was not surprised to find myself on a journey to such places. I didn't know why I had to go, just that I must. And likewise I knew I would make the flight to Inverness.

We choose how we want to experience life, and create it accordingly. Why was I employed on this journey? I didn't know. However, something was to happen, and I had to be there to let it happen.

As the taxi pulled up to the Findhorn Foundation, I felt nervous and alone, not knowing anyone. I glanced at the building known as Cluny Hill, where I would stay for the coming week. It seemed a bit run-down, I thought. Originally built as a grand hotel, it then became a spa, and now it was this college, part of the Findhorn Foundation. Nervously I climbed out of the cab, grabbed my bags, and headed toward the front door. There were people scattered everywhere. Some sat alone on the lawn sunning themselves, others laughed warmly in small groups as they sipped tea. Two men hugged each other. Another woman meditated as she faced the sun. I wondered why I had come, because I wasn't like these people — or was I? It was obvious to me that this was not normal society. Could it be too much, I wondered. My thoughts overwhelmed me.

After finding my room, I discovered I would have not one but two roommates. They were not there, but I could see by their luggage that they had already arrived. That made me a bit uneasy. I quickly unpacked and hid my valuables, not knowing if I could trust them. There was an hour before our group was to meet, so I went to the dining room and had some tea. It calmed me to sit and watch and listen to the many languages spoken. A cross-section of humanity from all parts of the world was there: black, yellow, white, old, middle-aged and young. They wore city shoes, birkenstocks, sandals and sneakers. My mind raced: Who will be in my group? Will I like them? Are they as crazy as I am to have come to this place?

As I gazed out over the beautiful golf course next door, the view of the hilly manicured greens inspired me. I sensed the inner beauty of the spirit of Findhorn and the openness of all who are there, and of all that have been there before. The warmth of their smiles was the first thing I noticed. They were genuine smiles, full of love. Everyone was equal. Everyone had their own gifts to share. Findhorn has none of the restraints that control people in society. Barriers such as color, creed, religion, sex and social bias are erased.

My heart beat quickly as I walked into our designated room to meet the others in my group for the first time. I sat nervously and glanced quickly at the other people. Who are my roommates, I wondered. Our group was large, we were nineteen. Malin had told me she had eight people in her group, and so I was surprised at the size of ours. But it was August, and many people were free for holidays. Our leader, Neils, was blessed with an incredible sense of caring and tenderness. He asked us to share brief introductions and tell what had brought us to Findhorn. In an intimate circle we sat and told from what country we came. I truly felt a love and warmth for everyone there. We were a cross-section of the world, and my two roommates were no exception. One was a Japanese child psychologist from Tokyo, and the other a land-surveyor from Belfast.

Many European countries were represented. As the introductions neared the end of the circle, there were three people who were directly across from me who had yet to introduce themselves. They each stated their names and home countries.

"I'm Jan-Helge from Norway."

"I'm Britt from Norway."

"I'm Grete from Norway."

How was it possible that I had never met a Norwegian, and yet I was preparing to embark on an intensive week with three people from there? Jan-Helge and Britt are a couple in a partnership, and Grete is a long-standing friend of theirs. They had made the excursion from Norway together. In awe, I listened as they talked briefly about themselves. They spoke English well, but it was obvious that it was not their primary language.

It was true, I realized as I gazed deep into their eyes. I felt a closeness with all of them, and tears came into my eyes when I looked into Grete's. There was a purpose for me to be in the same group as these three people from Norway. We had all selected the same week. After our group's introductions, I met the Norwegians.

"I had a map made for me that clearly showed that Norway has a strong energy for me. Does it for you?"

"For us, yes it does." Britt spoke for the other two, but they readily agreed.

They listened with great interest as I told them about my astrocartography map.

"You must visit our country one day so you can feel it for yourself!" Jan-Helge added.

Neils asked the group to join hands to meditate and tune in to each other. Nervously I looked around the room to see the reactions of the others as we began this first exercise. What did the rest of them think? I was open for anything, yet had no idea what to expect. We were told that when we tuned in, or centered ourselves, we needed to close our eyes while experiencing our concentrated energies. As we held hands, I became aware of not only myself, but also all the others with me. I felt something going around and around like the spinning of a top. Electricity surged through my body as an energy came into me from both sides of the circle. Overwhelmed, I recognized that this simple step was merely the beginning.

After this initial meeting, Neils guided us on a tour of the stately building and lush grounds to show us our new home for the week. During our tour, Britt happened to be in front of me. We stopped momentarily to listen to instructions on the use of the laundry facilities.

"Tim, I can feel your energy," Britt exclaimed as she turned to face me.

"My energy?"

"Yes."

Astonished, I gave a nervous half-laugh and asked, "Is it good?"

She smiled warmly and in her Norwegian-accented English asserted, "It is very good. I cannot always feel it on people, but it is good."

No one had ever told me such a thing. What exactly could she feel? I had only just met her and she had told me she was a holistic healer. Later that evening I sat drinking a cup of tea with the three of them.

"Perhaps we have all known each other before," Britt

offered.

I hesitated. "Before . . . what?"

"Before this life," she said. "And maybe we have been brought together to be recharged, and all for a reason that is yet unknown to us."

Not necessarily believing that birth is the beginning and death the end, I still didn't know what happens to us after we die.

She added, "We'll come to understand those reasons shortly."

Did she know something that I didn't? It was only the first day.

Behind the main building is a hill, the top of which is called the Power Point. There is a long winding walk to the top and I went there to reflect for an hour on that first day. As I sat I could feel a vibration, like a humming inside me. I thought of a cat, and how it purrs when it is at peace. That is what I felt. Findhorn is not the Garden of Eden, but the tranquillity helped me to feel what a paradise can be like when a sense of harmony prevails.

Yamaguchi and Paudge were my roommates. They were polite and I felt comfortable to share a space with them. The first night I was exhausted, and was ready to sleep. We said good night and turned out the lights. Yamaguchi drifted off at once and started to snore. Paudge and I tried to ignore it, but Yamaguchi snored louder and louder by the minute. I attempted to cover my ears, count sheep, and feign sleep to myself. After an hour or so I began to laugh, wondering how he could sleep — I thought he would wake himself up with his thunderous snoring. Never in my life had I heard such big sounds come out of such a little man. The next morning Paudge and I agreed that something had to be done before that evening. It would be a lesson in how to broach what could be a sensitive subject in a diplomatic manner to a virtual stranger. Yamaguchi felt bad that we had not slept. We mutually agreed that Paudge and I would sleep on mattresses in another room. It was important we rested well, and we did.

On Sunday morning we went to the sanctuary, a meditation chapel. We were asked to select our transformation or angel cards for the week. I laughed to myself as I wondered: Angel cards? What are they? Neils told us that angel cards represent something we need specifically to be aware of. They are almost always on target with what our souls need to work on. I drew my card. It was Faith. Pictured were two angels who swung on a trapeze — two people who are only successful if they work in unison. There was no question that I needed to have more faith in myself and in those with whom I shared my life.

I felt very comfortable with Neils. When I had a question, he was always responsive.

"Neils, I'm curious about meditation."

"Yes?"

"I know that when I meditate, I feel better inside."

"Yes."

"So if we meditate with thoughts directed toward someone specific, can they feel it? And therefore do they feel better too?"

"Yes, it is possible for anyone to feel what we send," Neils answered thoughtfully. "However, it depends on how sensitive they are. Some people don't want to receive anything from anyone, and therefore close themselves off. But those who are open, whose hearts and souls are open, yes, they can feel it."

On our second day, we were told we would all have work assignments for the week. Initially I thought to myself that I was on holiday, and did not want to work while there. However it was explained to us that the work projects are also a part of the total experience. Meals always need to be cooked, laundry needs to be done, and cleaning needs to take place. We sat in our circle as the different work assignments were explained. When I heard there was a gardening option, I decided that would be the one for me, because, not being very domestic, I didn't want to cook or clean.

We were asked to close our eyes and become as centered as possible, and we would decide by attunement. After a few moments' meditation, Neils said he would announce the list of jobs that needed to be filled, and how many people were required for each assignment. He said we would feel something inside ourselves for the job that would be ours for the week as he verbally listed them. My eyes were closed — I was ready to feel for the gardening job. The list was long. The fourth job he announced was for two people to help cook lunches in Cluny kitchen. I didn't understand what happened, but something inside me said, *Yeah — that's it*. It wasn't a voice, more a feeling, but I knew it was true. My mind said no, while my heart said yes.

When finally the gardening position was announced I felt absolutely nothing. After the list was read, we opened our eyes. Neils asked us to raise our hands for the jobs we sensed would be for us as he re-read the assignments so he could write down who would be doing what. When he announced "Two people for Cluny kitchen," I raised my hand along with only one other person, Sabine from Vienna, who became my friend. We were nineteen in our group, yet only two of us had sensed for the two posts in Cluny kitchen!

Dumbfounded at the accuracy of such a decision-making

system, I witnessed attunement used successfully over and over as Findhorn has perfected it to an art-form. Whether it is a problem to resolve, or a new avenue to venture forward on, they attune to feel the best direction in which to proceed. We were told it is also effective when we feel we may want to give to someone. No matter where we are in the world, be it New York, London, or rural India, we meet people with outstretched hands. It is impossible to give to everyone, but if we attune to those asking for help, we will feel for those specific individuals and react accordingly. It would be amazing if people all over the world could learn to listen to the voices in their hearts and souls instead of only the ones in their heads.

My experience in Cluny kitchen was incredible. Our leader, Elvira, was a beautiful woman. Her positive attitude made a strong impact on me. Whether we stirred salad dressing, diced onions, or scoured pots, she would walk by and invariably say, "Great!" By the time lunch was served every day I could not help but feel good because of her constant affirmations that the jobs we did were great. After a few days it amused me that no matter what we did, she was supportive. I realized how one little word — great — spoken with feeling, enthusiasm, trust and sincerity, had affected my whole experience. I decided to implement that word more often in my vocabulary, knowing if it made that much of an impact on me, then certainly it would on others around me. My inner spirit had been right about working in the kitchen.

On Monday Neils announced we would play games. Initially I felt frustrated when I heard this. Why do we have to play games? However, our recreation was multidimensional, and I soon learned I had jumped to the wrong conclusion. We began with simple exercises that helped us learn each other's names. Our scope then widened as the process evolved.

The games ranged from team and image playing, to trusting, to reflecting, to touch-feeling games. We played some with our eyes open, some with them closed. The experience was beautiful.

We were told at Findhorn to pay special attention to our dreams if we could remember them. I knew that our dreams are our subconscious talking to us. If we can tune in to our subconscious mind through dreaming, we will have a clearer understanding of the message for us in our daily conscious life.

By Tuesday morning, I had already had three dreams in which Norway was the predominant theme I remembered when I awakened. The dreams were too cloudy to recall details, but I clearly recognized in all three that I was in Norway. As a result, every morning my first conscious thought was about Norway. My subconscious had continually sent messages in my sleep, but I did not understand the meaning.

As the week progressed, I noticed a person that I felt drawn to. Our paths rarely crossed except at meal times because he was involved in another course. His shoulder-length wavy brown hair, his whiskers he called a beard, his brightly-colored clothing, his whole demeanor was completely the opposite of mine. He seemed so free and open. The clarity in his eyes was striking, and I knew when he smiled that it came from the depths within. I have always been fairly conservative and more reserved with my feelings and emotions. Yet there was something about his soul that drew mine. I felt an overwhelming desire to know him.

One day at lunch, we both were at the soup tureen at the same time.

"Hi, I don't know why, but I feel I need to meet you. My name is Tim."

He smiled and replied, "My name is Daniel."

My heart pounded. I felt nervous about making such a bold introduction.

"Where are you from?" I had heard him speak German, but his English was flawlessly American.

"Germany."

"That's incredible — you have no German accent."

"Thanks. My family lived in the States for two years when I was a kid, and I learned there."

We talked for only a few moments after that and spoke briefly only one other time that week. Glad to have met him, I instinctively knew we were kindred spirits, but I had no idea how strange an impact our meeting would have on me later.

The positive energy in the classes, meditations, work projects and social times inspired me. Experience Week is extremely intensive and emotionally exhausting. As a result, through the work we did, my inner focus began to rise to a higher plane than I have ever felt before. More whole, independent and centered, I was full of a vigorous new energy.

Midway through our week we had a group project to clean out and weed one of the beautiful gardens that surround Cluny Hill. I wondered what we would learn from weeding, as I had accepted the idea that all of our activities had a reason behind them. We often did not understand the purpose until later, but it was always made clear. As we weeded, we were instructed to put the short-rooted weeds in a compost pile, from which fertilizer would be made. The long-rooted weeds needed to be placed on a separate pile to be burnt, as they did not break down easily in a compost mixture. The ashes from that pile would then be spread around the garden. Therefore we used even the ugly weeds to work effectively, albeit in a different form. Easy enough, I thought. I busily weeded next to my friend Sandy.

"Tim," she remarked in her London cockney accent, "all your weeds have short roots, and so yours are easier to pull out. Look at mine, they are all long-rooted!"

It was true. Her section did have more long-rooted weeds, and she struggled individually with each one to pull them out. Suddenly she stopped, with a look of amazement in her eyes.

"Tim, this is my life — my roots are so deep. And they are ugly, deep weeds, not flowers! They are so hard to pull out. They are like my problems."

"Yeah, Sandy, but look, you're doing it, you are pulling them out!"

Little by little she made headway with her section. My weeds, my problems, were not quite as deep; however they were plentiful. Even though the project was a sweaty and dirty experience because we were in the garden, I felt good about my task as I understood the symbolism.

As I pulled a weed out of the ground, I saw a golf ball resting next to a flower. There is only a hedge that separates the garden from the golf course, so I was not surprised to find it there. I reached down and picked it up.

"I found a golf ball!" I yelled to my friends.

Grete walked by at that moment with a load of weeds for the compost pile. "Put it in your pocket and keep it as a souvenir. I just found one too!"

Having no affection for the sport of golf, I momentarily thought there was no reason I would want to save a golf ball. However, I reconsidered because I was at Findhorn.

After deciding it would be a good memento of my experience in the garden, I placed it in my pocket and continued to weed. When we finished the project, we returned our buckets and gloves to the greenhouse.

"Tim, may I see your golf ball?" Grete asked at the tool shed.

What an odd request, I thought. All golf balls look alike to me: they are small, white, round, with tiny dimples all over, and usually have some numbers and a company logo printed on them. Why did she want to see mine? It looked just like hers. She had her golf ball in her hand, and offered it to me to look at. I pulled mine out from my pocket, glanced at it, and handed it to her. Then I inspected hers and noted her golf ball did have a different logo and even different numbers than mine.

"Do you know what 332 is?" she asked after she had looked at mine for a few moments.

The numbers 332 were printed on the face of my golf ball.

"No, what is it?"

"332 is my house address."

"Your address?" I fumbled with my words. "Of your home in Norway?"

"Yes." She smiled.

I double-checked her golf ball that was still in my hand. Her numbers were different from mine.

"Grete, what do you think this means?"

She grinned. "It means whatever you want it to mean."

Beneath the stamped 332 on my golf ball was another number, 4.

"What does 4 stand for?"

"The number 4 is destiny," she explained to me.

I swallowed. In numerology all numbers have a specific significance. Britt and Jan-Helge happened to be nearby, and so I handed them my golf ball.

"Look what I found with Grete's address," I said to them shyly, knowing somehow there was a deeper significance that was soon to be revealed to me.

They both chuckled as they confirmed it was indeed Grete's house number. I couldn't help but think that 332 was an odd set of digits to be printed on a golf ball.

After the garden weeding project I went to the midday meditation. It was in the same sanctuary where I had heard the most beautiful singing earlier that morning. The walls still seemed to echo the Gregorian-Buddhist chanting.

Sitting comfortably I closed my eyes. Immediately I recognized my mind was taking me on a journey. From another level of consciousness I could clearly see an image of Grete and myself seated side by side on an airplane, and I knew the plane was destined for Norway. Then, I saw myself meditating on top of a mountain. Again, it was clear to me that I was in Norway. The panorama that materialized in my vision astonished me. Spread below me out to the horizon were lush green hills, a city shining in the sun, and brilliant azure water as it flowed into the fjords, and all the while the ocean hovered in the background in its deep blue vastness. The image seemed a fantasy. I had never been to Norway, nor had any idea what it looked like, but I had figuratively just seen a part of it as if I gazed upon a beautiful painting in a museum. It was as though I observed another reality, yet in my own space and time.

After about twenty minutes in the sanctuary, I left and immediately bumped into Britt. Overwhelmed, I had to explain to her what I had just seen. She smiled.

"There is a mountain directly behind Grete's house that we all frequently climb to meditate on the top," she said. "The mountain overlooks all of Bergen, our city."

My eyes filled with tears.

"I was just there," I whispered. "It was as clear as the view through an open window, and it was beautiful. Britt, what should I do?"

"You must go to Norway with Grete," she answered with a soothing yet matter-of-fact tone to her voice.

I breathed in deeply, exhaling long and slow. "What do I do when I get there?"

"Don't worry about that," she reassured me. "You'll find out when you arrive. Trust and have faith — there is nothing to be afraid of."

"But why did I see this?"

The question just came out, though I knew what she would tell me.

"You're experiencing different space-times, or parallel realities, to change your thinking — and your life."

Grete was outside and I went and told her what I had seen in my meditation.

"Tim, you can come home with me and you are welcome to stay as long as you feel you need to."

"Thanks," I said as we hugged. "I don't understand why, but I must go with you."

Jan-Helge and Britt had decided to stay on in Great Britain for a while, so Grete was to return alone. She had already gone once to try to buy her ticket, but had left in frustration. Between the travel agent's Scottish accent and Grete's Norwegian-inflected English, neither could understand the other. They had both spoken the same language to each other, but could not communicate. Grete needed me to interpret for her.

The next afternoon we found our way to the travel agency to buy our tickets. We were offered two options for travel to Norway. Besides the flight, there was also an overnight ferry across the North Sea between Scotland and Norway. It took much longer, but was more economical. For a moment I considered the ship option as I thought it might be a memorable experience to cross by water. Abruptly the image I had seen the day before reappeared in my mind.

"Grete, we have to fly," I urged as I remembered Grete and myself seated on an airplane — not on a ship.

"OK, so we fly, we'll get there fast, and we can spend time with Jan-Helge and Britt before we leave," Grete confirmed agreeably.

Our Experience Week would finish on Saturday, so we bought our tickets to leave the following Tuesday. Thus we could look forward to three days to relax and unwind in Scotland.

Overwhelmed at what had occurred in so short a period of time, I realized my every action and breath led effortlessly to the next. How could this happen to me, I wondered.

When I was still and listened to my inner self, I learned I would never be led astray. What seemed to be trivial coincidences proved to be quite significant. These incidents all had purpose and importance. I only needed to stop and listen to my inner voice and have faith. There was no concrete reason why I was pulled to go to Norway; my soul simply was drawn there. Who was I to doubt the events that had unfolded?

At Thursday morning's breakfast of healthy whole-wheat bread, fruit and tea, Sandy and I were involved in conversation. She sat on my left. I could not turn all the way to the left to see her because I had a kink in my neck. Nor could I turn to the right. I complained to her of my ailment.

"Sandy, can you massage my neck a bit?"

"Sure, but why can't you look left or right?"

"It's my pillow," I naively explained. "It's harder than what I normally sleep on. The last two nights I woke up with the same problem."

"You really believe that?"

Confused, I responded, "Yeah," as I could conceive of no other explanation. Thus began my introduction to metaphysics.

"Tim," Sandy disputed with a twinkle in her eye, "you're at Findhorn. You are facing many issues you have never confronted before. Do you think your inability to see to the left or right has anything to do with the fact that there are aspects of your emotional/female or intellectual/male side that you don't want to confront?"

Her challenge gave me reason to pause and think. It was not normal for me to develop kinks in my neck. Many stranger realizations had hit me during the week, and so I was open to what Sandy had to say. Metaphysics is the study of what is outside the objective experience. It is a theoretical approach to philosophy that can never be verified. I certainly could not prove my kinks as the fault of the pillow, nor could I imagine them as being caused by my unwillingness to face a part of me I was afraid to see. Yet I knew Sandy had opened a door in my life that shed a new light.

Friday night heralded our final sharing, meditation, and celebration dinner together. In our last exchange, we each had the opportunity to thank the others and observe how we had grown during the week. It was scheduled to be a two-hour session. Four and a half hours later, after much laughter, many tears, and the deepest of sharing, we had finished. Through my many realizations, I saw how untrusting I had been on my arrival when I had hidden my valuables from my roommates. I had been very mistaken.

They were two beautiful people, and even through Yamaguchi's snoring, when I looked at him I could only feel love. Cluny Hill had become my home, too. It was sad to leave that old building that held so much life. My thoughts flashed back to how I had considered it old and run-down when I arrived.

The map I had been given a few weeks earlier had become the road map of my journey into awareness and transformation. I had felt the powers of Scotland, and was soon to be on my way to Norway.

I pondered how the entire world might improve if we could all share this generous level of unconditional love and compassion. We had naturally become as family to each other in a mere seven days. However, in our final meeting we could feel our group's energy begin to dissipate. We then understood that the appropriate time to leave Findhorn had come. Just the day before, none of us could imagine leaving. I knew it was over, but I wasn't sad. As safe and warm as it was at Cluny Hill, we knew we could not linger there forever — we understood it was time to move forward. Our life's journey was ready to re-commence. It was a beautiful understanding.

10

The Park

Midway through our Experience Week I realized I needed to find a place to stay from Saturday, when the program was over, until Tuesday, when Grete and I were to leave. On Wednesday, after I had found the golf ball, I thought to ask about reserving a room at Newbold House, a small community associated with the Findhorn Foundation which takes guests. However, I neglected to call, and blamed it on procrastination. Not until Friday evening did I inquire. They informed me they would be full for the weekend — literally no room at the inn. Should I have called earlier? What did it mean? Perhaps someone needed the bed more than I. Findhorn had taught me to listen to these silent messages.

Concerned about where to stay for the next few nights, I remembered my Norwegian friends had a camper that slept six people, yet I hesitated to ask them if I could stay for three days. However the thought occurred that perhaps I needed to spend time with all three of them. So I asked. They all responded agreeably; it would not be a problem. Jan-Helge and Britt shared a bed, Grete had a bed, and I could sleep in the third bed. I felt relieved. They parked their camper over at the Park. The Park is another integral part of the Findhorn Foundation, a few miles distant from Cluny Hill. A majority of the people who work at Findhorn live at the Park. It includes a hall used for performances, meetings and theatrical productions, a campground for trailers and tents, a community center with dining hall, a bookstore, and the administration buildings.

The camper became my home when I moved my bags in. It was a communal life: fun, clean and natural, and I was surrounded by three extraordinary friends. The air was full of acceptance and love. I felt as though something was to happen. What destiny was I to follow, I wondered, as I pondered the number 4 on my golf ball. Somehow I knew I had much to do.

Saturday, the first day at the Park, I napped three times. Emotionally exhausted, my physical body needed and craved sleep. The intensity of the previous week's activities had caught up with me. A week at Findhorn seemed like a year. So much had transpired in so short a period of time. We were all beyond any normal state of fatigue — it was sheer exhaustion.

Originally I had planned to tour the area around Inverness during my three days' rest between the Experience Week and departing for Norway. The infamous Loch Ness is nearby, and I had been captivated by its mystery since I was a small child. However, I had no energy to contemplate any sort of physical trek. I found humor in the fact I was so near that famous loch, but could not muster the desire to go there. Content to stay at the Park, all I wanted was to rest and recharge myself.

Residents and guests alike at the Park frequently gather and mingle at the café. Saturday evening I walked there to see if any others from our group had also migrated to the Park. Instead I ran right into that long-haired German with whiskers and red jeans.

"Daniel!"

"Hey Tim, I was wondering about you."

"Me too."

"I've just realized that when I left Cluny Hill I didn't say goodbye to some of the people I'd met."

"So we meet again!"

"It's funny," he said thoughtfully, "people come into and out of our lives so fast sometimes. When I meet strangers

I ask myself what their purpose is for me — or what is mine for them. You're one of them."

We sat on a large boulder with a little pond underneath in the twilight of early evening. Several small children played and giggled in the water at our feet. There was a sing-along happening inside the open doors of the café, so we easily overheard the songs and accompanying laughter. The various participants sang or played their harmonicas and guitars.

"I know the feeling," I said. "When you part, you wonder when you'll see your friends again. This life — or the next? I wondered about you too. So we run into each other again. Do you believe we're guided?"

"Sure, we're all guided aren't we?"

"Yes, but for what, to go where?"

"To learn."

"Yeah, to learn something," I repeated.

"Who is your teacher?"

"Well, we have many teachers as we go."

"Yeah, but who is your teacher?"

We both laughed as we played with each other's thoughts.

"I guess I am."

"And I'm my own too?"

"Sure."

It's all so simple. We realized we could talk like this for hours, each probing, pushing the other to think, to feel.

"Two or three times last week when I looked into your eyes I felt I wanted to know you, talk to you," Daniel said. "But it's so hard to mix with people from other groups. There was no time."

My words came from my heart. "To be honest, I felt the same about you. When I left Cluny Hill, I thought that there was someone inside that guy named Daniel that I wanted to know. Of course I assumed I'd never see you again. And here you are taking a walk like me. I just came over here myself — I'm staying in a camper with three friends who were in my group. Where are you staying?"

"There's a little bed and breakfast I found here, it's perfect for what I need."

The sky was clear, but as the sun set, the cool evening forced us to button up. The children who had been playing at our feet were called inside by their mothers. Suddenly we were alone on the rock.

"So what will you do now?" I asked.

"I need to rest and do nothing. I've been here two weeks — I did Experience Week One and then Two, back to back. It was overwhelming for me, not that I regret it, but it was almost too much for me to do without a break between the two. Eventually though, before I go back to Berlin next Saturday, I will travel around in England. Stonehenge and the stone circles at Avebury are on my list."

"Wow."

"And you? What will you do?"

I laughed. "Well, some incredible things have happened to me, and as a result I leave for Norway with one of my Norwegian friends on Tuesday."

"Oh! Tell me."

"Well, it is a good story . . ."

Naturally I had to explain to him that I was going to Norway because I had found a golf ball. We laughed together. It is a strange reason to go somewhere. I knew he could understand.

He asked me about my family and I about his. We slowly began to get acquainted. The feeling was that we somehow already knew all the answers to the questions we asked. It was as though we had always been friends, or known each other. We both admitted that we felt a close kinship. Our connection was strong.

"What would you think if I shaved my beard?"

He felt it made him look older. I thought it made him look scruffy.

"Yeah, you'd look good," I responded.

"OK, it comes off tonight!"

That evening my friends from Norway shared with me their tradition of drinking hot water. It cleanses the body they told me. OK. Quickly adapting to their custom, I began to drink hot water in earnest. Our conversations seemed always to be serious. For example, frequently they were in-depth discourses on our gifts of *light* that we all knew we shared. We spoke further of our gifts of power, love and intuition. But the subject of light bore the most interest for me. The type of person who lives in the light lives with a mind open to mental, emotional and spiritual evolution.

"Tim, we are light," Britt said. "The light is not outside of us; rather, it is within."

"It's easy to see others who have light," Grete continued, "because they have an inner radiance. They stay in tune with who they are."

Jan-Helge was next: "There are people who live their lives in brightness and are happy, but there are many more who choose to be discouraged and figuratively live in the dark."

"People choose to be unhappy?" I asked.

"Absolutely," replied Britt.

"We're all in control and we live our lives the way we want," Jan-Helge added.

Grete was lying down, her head propped up on her arm. Her eyes radiated the same clarity as her spoken thoughts. "We choose our experiences based on what lessons our souls need to learn."

"We choose our lessons?" I tried to understand. "So this is all our choice?"

"Yes, everyone makes their own choices."

"Hmmm."

"Tim, many people do not realize it, but we all have control over what we do and how we live out our lives."

"So I must let everyone else be, because that is how they choose to be?"

"Exactly."

Slowly I made progress. "And also, I am how I choose to be? Or, I am how I allow myself to be?"

"Yes!" they all exclaimed as they realized I had suddenly walked through another light-filled doorway.

"But you are not just how you choose to be," continued Grete, "but also who, what and where — you have chosen it all."

"Tim, you have light within. I saw it, I felt it, when I met you," Britt said. "With your positive outlook toward life, I know you are in complete control. You're not driving blindly. Because of your light, your soul has guided you — you know where you are going."

"Where am I going?"

"Feel it in your soul!"

It was like pulling petals off a rose, and slowly getting to visualize the center of it.

"Everything is OK," Grete added, "because we are all here for different reasons. Some souls have more to accomplish than others."

Jan-Helge continued, "There are many people who don't want to do any more than what they let their life deliver to them. They allow themselves to be sad, angry, even hateful. We can meditate for them, pray for them, send them our energy. But their drama is not our drama. We need to practice acceptance of all. That is compassion."

Talking aloud as I processed my thoughts, I said: "So I chose to be born in Orlando in 1961?"

"Yes."

"Further, I also chose my parents and family for the lessons I need to learn from them?"

"Bravo — but also for the lessons they need to learn from you."

"And I have chosen every experience that I have lived thus far?"

"Yes — including being here with us right now!"

That evening I slept soundly. Sunday morning I was the first to awaken and I quietly left the camper for some breakfast in the community center. A little while later, Daniel arrived. He looked depressed — I knew something was not right when he asked for a long hug.

"What happened?"

"Just hold me a minute, I need some love," he said.

The dining room was full and I glanced around, wondering if anyone was watching us. Then I realized no one cared.

"Tim, let's get a cup of tea and sit down."

"OK."

"The woman who owns the bed and breakfast where I stayed last night sent a messenger this morning to tell me that I must leave."

"Why?"

"I don't understand," he said. "The messenger alleged the owner had an occasional problem with men, but why would someone here have a problem with a Foundation guest?"

"Did you ever talk with the owner?"

"Yes, but only for a minute when I checked in. Last night

I didn't get in until late — because I was talking with you. When I woke up this morning, I did my yoga in the yard, and that's when the messenger came."

"Maybe she's afraid of men with long hair," I offered. "Did she see you without a beard — because you look good by the way."

He did look more clean-cut without the beard.

He grinned. "Thanks, I thought the beard made me look older, but I feel better without it. Where are you staying?"

Daniel had never met my Norwegian friends. I told him that if the camper were mine, I would not care if he stayed with us; however the camper was not mine, I was a guest. We spoke for a while and he was able to relax.

"I wonder what this means. There must be a reason behind my getting kicked out."

"Yeah, I'm learning myself that there's always another explanation to things like this. We'll see what happens."

He confessed he felt better after talking through his temporary troubles.

"Can I meet your friends?" he asked. "If they don't have a place for me, maybe they know of someone who might."

As we walked to the camper, I felt nervous to ask them if a fifth party could move in with us — especially someone they did not know.

Jan-Helge, Britt and Grete were awake and at the table with their mugs of hot water. We happily joined in and briefly shared introductions. Though Daniel had been in a different group than ours the week before, we all recognized we had the same Findhorn background of truth and honesty.

"Ahhh, you're the one who had a beard last week," said Britt.

"Now we can see who that man is who was behind it!" Jan-Helge remarked as he joined in.

As we all laughed I realized Daniel had quickly been adopted as part of our family on wheels. None of them hesitated when he asked to move into the camper. It seemed so natural, as if it were part of the plan.

Daniel was free, loose and uninhibited. I, on the other hand, always felt more structured and regimented with my life — yet there was something that drew me to him. He was ten years younger than I, perhaps I simply yearned to be more youthful. Frightened to feel any sort of attraction to him, I was confused by my feelings.

In the cool hours of early evening Daniel and I donned heavy sweaters and strolled into Findhorn village for dinner. As we were in Scotland, fish and chips seemed an appropriate meal. We found an outdoor restaurant that overlooked the bay. We watched the fishermen wade slowly through the marshy flats. Islands of clumped reeds grew high and we could easily see the muddy byways created by the ebb tide.

Our time in Scotland until then had been spent solely with people from the Foundation. We thought it a good idea to acclimatize ourselves back into normal society, so we enjoyed ourselves in a public restaurant. We spoke in more detail of our personal lives — he of his present relationship with a woman, and I of my past relationship with a man. We both had curious and fun questions to put to each other. Daniel shared with me some of the sexual confusion that he had been facing in the past few years. He had always been curious about men who were in relationships with men. However he had been afraid to confront that particular possibility for himself until he met me.

"I have something to tell you," Daniel said.

"Yeah?"

"Every time I saw you last week, I was really aware of how I looked."

I smiled. "Why?"

"I don't know, I just wanted to look good in front of you."

"You don't strike me as the type of person who cares what other people think about how you look."

"Well, I don't. But I did with you. I laughed to myself every time I saw you because these thoughts came to mind."

"So what did you do?" I asked.

"I didn't do anything to myself — I just hoped I looked good when I saw you."

"And now look what happened — we're having dinner!" I wondered why we had been brought together.

We laughed and ate as the northern Scottish sun set low over the horizon. Time flew quickly.

"Something's happening," I said.

"I know! But what?"

"I don't know!"

We both had learned the beauty of the concept 'Findhorn honesty'. That is to say, if we communicate our true feelings to the person with whom we share, be they positive or negative, then our communication will be pure and honest.

"Daniel, you know tonight we will be sleeping in the same bed in the camper."

"Yeah."

"Well, I need to tell you that I'm glad."

"Oh."

"Does that make you nervous?"

He laughed. "No, but it seems to make you nervous to tell me."

"Well yes, maybe just a little — or maybe more than a little . . ."

We both laughed as we walked back toward the Park.

"I just felt I needed to share that with you before we get back. I don't want you to be uncomfortable."

"If you're OK with it, then I am too."

In an odd way his strength gave me strength.

"There is a certain energy that is passed from body to body in the sleeping process that soothes the spirit between two people who care for each other," I said. "So I suppose what I'm telling you is that I care for you, like I've known you forever."

"Thanks, that really makes me feel good."

After our dinner we again became immersed in heavy conversation with our Norwegian friends. Jan-Helge had decided it was time for a bit of Findhorn honesty.

"Britt, I'm feeling uncomfortable with you because whenever we are all together in a group, you give Tim more attention in our conversations than you give to anyone else."

Boom! Suddenly a lead balloon had descended upon me. I felt horrible, as if everything was my fault. My mind raced as I tried to imagine what I could do to alleviate the problem. I hated situations like this — and now I found myself in the center of one. There was silence. Grete and Daniel didn't say a word. After several moments Britt responded.

"Yes, Jan-Helge, I can understand what you are saying."

The two of them then talked for a while about old patterns that had arisen — patterns they wanted to erase from their lives. The three of us listened and learned.

"Tim, you must know this is not your fault or doing," Britt assured me. "You have come into our group, and one of the lessons I must learn I have learned because of you. Thank you."

I gulped. Thank you? Honesty was tough. Jan-Helge was straight and to the point; his intimate frankness had been difficult to hear. However, the exercise served to strengthen both of them because they understood the purpose. They were able to resolve their differences quickly, as they had worked through this truth process on many occasions. We learned that we are all responsible for the negative and positive events that constantly flow through our lives. If we can be honest with each other, and more importantly with ourselves, then all obstructions will fall away. As problems are faced and acknowledged, they will be resolved. I began to understand why the five of us had been brought together. We had many lessons to learn from each other.

On Monday morning, Daniel and I arose earlier than the others and left the camper to do yoga and have some tea. As he showed me how he did his morning yoga routine, he shared some of his feelings.

"Tim, two or three times last night I woke up out of fear."

"Why?"

"Because I was asleep next to a man."

"And, so?"

"Well, every time I awoke, I realized there was nothing to be afraid of, and fell back asleep."

"So are you OK now?"

He laughed. "Of course. I have this thing with fear. It tends to get in my own way a lot!"

"So as long as we're being honest, it was nice for me to sleep next to you. Not from a sense of longing, but because of an intimate sense of companionship. Thanks."

He smiled. "No problem."

We shared our feelings of having been at Findhorn forever, and of having known each other for an eternity, when in reality only 24 hours had gone by.

"Daniel, what time is it?"

"I have no idea."

"Do you know what day it is?"

"Do you?"

"No!"

We had to laugh. Time did not advance according to the

clock, the way society had taught us. It somehow sped up, and we joked constantly as we wondered what day, month, and even what year it was. We had lost all concept of time. It then occurred to me, after working out what day it was, that Grete and I were to fly to Norway the next morning.

After our yoga, Daniel and I returned to the camper. Our friends were drowsily awake and at the table with their hot water.

"Daniel, I think tomorrow you will go to Norway with Tim and Grete," Britt said with a smile on her face. We all turned and stared at him.

Shocked, Daniel affirmed, "No, tomorrow I'm going south towards London."

Britt questioned him again, with a twinkle in her eye, saying, "Are you quite sure about that?"

"Yes," he said, though the expression on his face reflected his confusion.

"I think you will come with us too, Daniel," Grete added.

When I heard Britt's remark, it occurred to me that Daniel must come to Norway with us. Why, I did not know, not even for myself. However, Britt's intuitive comment sent a glimmer of truth through me. It was a moment when suddenly everything seemed clear, without being in any way understandable.

Daniel hesitantly half-laughed again, perhaps afraid they knew more about him and what he was about to do than he wished they did.

"No, tomorrow I'll be on my way to London!" he strongly reiterated. "I've never even thought about a trip to Norway, I don't have a ticket, and I can't change my travel plans so drastically and so fast. The flight is tomorrow morning!"

Michelle and I were flying. We laughed out loud and were very happy.

That was all I remembered of my dream the previous night when I had woken up actually laughing. Michelle was a good friend of mine in college who married my roommate. In the twelve years since I graduated, I could not remember ever dreaming about college. However, for the past six months I had had numerous dreams about a handful of good friends of mine from school. They were becoming more and more frequent, and I clearly remembered them. I always woke up feeling good. I asked Jan-Helge and Britt about it.

They told me that these dreams reflected a period in my life that, though over long ago, was very happy. My overall sense of calm and contentment now is like it was then. The dreams were always positive, with strong and good people in them. It was not uncommon for me to wake up laughing. Britt said I had worked hard in the years since college, and hadn't allowed myself to feel my own feelings. However, the dreams were a good indicator that reflected my changed outlook in my life in the past six months.

It was our final day, and we made our plans to leave. Grete and I needed to find the train station to purchase our tickets to Aberdeen. As Aberdeen was two hours away, and our flight left at 9:15 the next morning, we knew we must wake up early to catch the first train. Daniel came with Grete and me to the station to buy his ticket to London. As the three of us walked arm in arm through the warm sunny streets, we felt truly alive and in harmony with each other.

"Daniel, what will you do?" I asked.

Knowing well what I referred to, he affirmed, "I'm going to London!"

He again explained he was absolutely sure of his decision. I conceded to him that if that is how he truly felt inside, then he must go to London.

As we neared the station I began to feel nauseous. My eyesight became blurry, and I knew something was not right. The strength drained from my legs. I reached the window first and bought my train ticket to Aberdeen. Grete was next. Finally Daniel stepped up to the window. I could barely stand — it was overwhelming. Grete went into the bathroom and I had to sit on a bench near the bathroom door. From where I sat I could see Daniel as he spoke to the ticket agent. After two or three minutes of conversation, Daniel nervously wrote some figures on a piece of scratch paper; however he never pulled out any money. Grete came out of the bathroom and sat with me just as Daniel turned to come towards us.

"He can't buy a ticket can he?" Grete said.

I wondered how she knew. By then Daniel had returned to us, and with frustration told us what had happened.

"They won't sell me a ticket to London."

"Why not?" I asked.

"Because I want to stop in a few towns on the way, and take maybe three or four days to get there. I want to see Avebury, Stonehenge, and maybe some other places, but I haven't yet decided, and they will only sell a ticket to London, or a ticket to Glasgow, or a ticket to Newcastle, but I don't know where I want to get off until I get there. So I didn't buy a ticket. I don't know what to do."

Grete knew.

"Do you understand what this means?" she asked with a smile.

"This is too much!" he confessed in agony. "I don't want to think about it now, I'm hungry."

In his confusion, he chose not to acknowledge the silent

messages that were coming his way. He continued to assert that the next day he would be en route towards London. Physically weak and overwhelmed, I too wanted out of the station. For the first time in ten days I wasn't centered. When I am centered I feel an inner peace with myself. However, I wasn't in control of my mind or body. We ran out of the train station and hunted for a place to eat. We quickly found a diner, entered and sat down. Grete and Daniel then looked around, and jointly decided it was not the place for us.

"We can't leave now, " I protested, "it would be rude, we just got our water."

"Oh yes we can," Daniel and Grete responded in unison. "This place doesn't feel right."

A few doors down the street we found an Indian restaurant. Daniel had lived in India for a few months and loved Indian food. It was healthy and wholesome. He wasn't centered either; he needed to find balance from within. Indian food was something he knew, something familiar. The meal helped to ground him, and he felt better afterwards. Even I agreed the restaurant felt right. Grete and I enjoyed the opportunity to sit and sample new foods with Daniel as he guided us through the menu.

We needed to share and tune in, and back at the camper we had our opportunity. The three of us explained to Jan-Helge and Britt what had occurred at the train station.

"I am completely confused," I began to explain to my German and Norwegian friends at the table, "and there are four different possible reasons for this confusion. One, I don't know if perhaps I feel off base because Daniel is to go to London, and I have found that I am attracted to him; or two, that perhaps he needs to accomplish a mission like I do in Norway; or three, that Grete, Daniel and I all have something to do together in Norway; or four, a combination of any or all the above."

There, I had said it. Everything was out on the table. There were no secrets. I looked at Daniel and wondered if he was upset that I had shared with our friends what I felt about him. No, I could see he was not upset. In fact he just smiled at me. Grete then joined in.

"I feel an attraction to Daniel too," she confessed.

I could see she was shocked that I did as well.

"And in fact, Daniel, if you were ten years older, I would marry you."

"What's wrong with my age?" Daniel countered jokingly. "Why can't you marry me now?"

"You're too young," she explained.

Grete was 35, I was 34, and Daniel was 24.

A ten-minute discussion about age, and the difference it makes, then ensued between them. Jan-Helge and Britt sat across from us and listened with amusement. I was between the two of them, and getting redder by the minute. Finally I couldn't take any more.

"I started this conversation because I wanted to share what I felt towards Daniel," I announced, "and you two discuss marriage!"

Britt broke into laughter and with a chuckle said, "You three have a drama triangle!"

We all laughed. It was humorous, and the lightness helped relax us. We had a definite connection with each other, but none of us could yet understand what it was. Daniel was still confused about what decision to make.

Britt advised Daniel, "You need to meditate and relax, and feel what you want to do with your heart, not with your head."

"But I am trying to listen to my heart," he protested. "It's just my fear that pops up all the time."

"Your fear comes from your ego — not your heart. Listen

to your heart."

In the early evening we drove down to the Moray Firth, a tributary of the North Sea, to look for dolphins, many of which live in the area. Daniel and I spoke together on the shore of the bay.

"If you really feel in your heart you must go to London, then go. Know that I will support you in your feelings."

The waves chopped noisily while we relaxed into that serene peacefulness that is so easy to find by the sea. From one moment to the next Daniel's many doubts, fears and anxieties underwent a small transformation.

"I can't take any more of this," he declared in resignation. "I'm going with you!"

Stunned, I stared at him, not believing what he had just said. Then we hugged warmly.

"I hope I'm doing the right thing," he said.

"You are."

I knew he was. We walked back into the camper smiling from ear to ear.

"Did you see some dolphins?" they all asked, convinced by our faces that we had found what we were looking for.

"No, we didn't find the dolphins," Daniel explained, "but I did come to a big decision . . ."

They listened with rapt attention, wondering what he had to say. I just smiled.

"I'm going to Norway tomorrow with Tim and Grete!"

"Yahoo!" Everyone cheered their support. Jan-Helge, Britt, Grete and I exchanged huge grins.

"You made the right decision, Daniel," confirmed Britt.

"But what if I can't get on the plane tomorrow?" he said with a hint of fear in his voice. "What if it's sold out, what will I do?"

"If you are to go on this journey, there will be a seat for you," Britt responded calmly, "and you are to go, so don't worry."

How could she make such powerful and assertive statements, I thought. How does she know there will be a seat? Daniel contended he had never made a decision like that before in his life. He was surprised at himself, but was finally convinced that he must join Grete and me in Norway. He had to call his girlfriend, Tessa, in Berlin and tell her he would be on a plane to Norway the next day, and he had no idea how long he would be gone. He was visibly nervous about calling her. After talking to her, he came to us and asked for hugs and love because she was upset with him. We assured him his decision was right.

"Daniel, you must make your decisions in life based on what you feel you need to do, not on what others expect you to do," I said.

"It's not so much that Tessa pressures me — although sometimes I feel she does. It's more that I allow myself to feel pressured by her expectations."

David was in London waiting for me to call. I used the same phone booth.

"David — I'm not coming back right away to London. I found a golf ball, and so I'm going to Norway."

"What?"

The time on the phonecard was running out fast. I had only a few moments to talk.

"I'm going with a Norwegian woman and a guy from Germany."

"Why?"

"I have no idea. I'll find out when I get there."

"I don't understand the golf ball."

"Well it had Grete's address on it."

He humored me. "Ahhh, then that's OK."

Though David was stressed regarding some events that had transpired in his life, he shared my enthusiasm. He said he had sensed all through the week that something incredible was happening. I could hear in his voice that he yearned to have an experience like mine.

The phonecard ran out as he yelled, "Wait for me!"

The next morning we were up before the sun. Barely awake, we staggered aboard the 6:00 am train to Aberdeen. As we fumbled with our bags, we laughed in disbelief that we were now three people employed on this journey. Daniel still didn't know if he could get on the flight. We had all been thrown together through such curious twists of fate. At first we tried to analyze why, but realized it would be an impossible task. So we just accepted it, and let it be.

I was on my way to Norway. The astrologer three weeks before had strongly advised me to consider visiting it one day. What was the magnetic or mere suggestive power that drew me, and how did it work so effectively?

As the train neared Aberdeen, our airport stop went by unnoticed. When we realized our error we suffered a moment of great anxiety.

"Hey, that was our stop!" I exclaimed as the train pulled away from the station and I saw the airport runway in the background.

"What do we do?"

Time was of the essence. Somehow, though we had not spoken loudly, a young man across from us overheard our concerned voices. He volunteered information that proved invaluable.

"If you get off at the next stop and cross quickly to track eleven nearby, there will be a train leaving within one minute that returns to the airport. But you've got to run!"

Upon arrival, we dashed off the train, up the stairs and down to the correct track. We raced and made it!

On the return train, as we again neared the airport, another lady overheard our anxious conversation.

"Don't worry," she said, "there is always a bus and usually a taxi at the next stop that can take you to the airport terminal."

"Thanks."

I realized we hadn't asked anyone for assistance, but help and guidance were being offered to us at every turn.

We found a taxi straightaway. The driver was a kindly old Scot with a good sense of humor.

"Did you get hurt when you fell?" he queried.

None of us understood the question; we looked at each other with blank faces. His hardy accent was the standard Scottish brogue, and we had a difficult time understanding him. After a few silent moments, we realized his question was directed at Grete because he continued to look at her in the rear-view mirror. She was visibly confused, and did not know how to respond.

"Did you get hurt when you fell *from heaven*?" he added at last.

We burst into laughter when finally we understood that he was suggesting she was an angel. His wonderful sense of humor helped lighten our brief ride to the airport.

Because of our miscalculation on the train, we didn't get to the terminal until 8:45. The flight left at 9:15, and Daniel was without a ticket. We ran inside only to hear that our flight had been canceled. However, they had rescheduled all the passengers onto another flight that was to leave within a few minutes. Because Grete and I had our tickets, we only needed to check in. There seemed to be a lot of confusion in the terminal, because we repeatedly received conflicting directions as to where to buy an additional ticket. It was a race against time. Our hearts pounded in anxiety. Daniel asked me to stay by his side, as he was concerned he might lack enough British pounds to buy his ticket. I had earlier volunteered to help pay the balance if he needed it. We finally found the correct ticket agent.

"I need one ticket to Bergen on the flight that leaves in 15 minutes," I stated.

"Why are you so late?" the agent screamed.

"Because we just got here!"

She frantically typed onto the computer console. She was visibly nervous herself. The clock on the wall behind her continued to tick steadily onward, oblivious to our desire to stop it for a few minutes. Finally she looked up.

"There is only one seat left on that flight."

I glanced at Daniel. He had the most incredulous expression on his face.

"We'll take it!" I affirmed loudly.

"Wait! How much is it?" cried Daniel. "I have an I.D. card that proves I'm under 25 if that helps."

Anyone under 25 in Europe has the privilege of flying for greatly reduced fares. He showed her the card. Grete and I had each paid £240. Daniel had only £180. One of his fears had been the possibility he would not have enough money to get to Norway.

She typed some more information onto the keyboard. "That seat is £106."

The flight was to leave in 10 minutes. She printed out his ticket, he threw her the money, and laughing the three of us sprinted through the airport to catch our flight. We had only a few moments to spare and were the last ones to board. We found our assigned seats — Grete was by the window and I was next to her. Across the aisle from me was the last available seat on the flight, and Daniel was the occupant. He sat next to a middle-aged woman. We sighed a breath of relief. Through what seemed invincible odds, we were all together on the way to Norway.

As I sat catching my breath, I looked forward into the plane and shuddered. I grabbed and held Grete's hand.

"Grete, this is exactly what I saw when I meditated last week." I stared with disbelief at the cabin of the airplane. "You and I were sitting right here — just like this!"

After the plane took off, I asked Daniel to stand and look forward to confirm if there were any empty seats. There were none.

En route Grete expressed to me one of her grave fears. "Norway," she explained, "is a very conservative country. I am nervous to go home from my vacation with two foreign men. I'm afraid of what my neighbors will think, and what my two young sons will say."

She had been divorced for a few years.

"The boys have been in Denmark all summer with their father, and will come home tonight."

She was anxious because the three of us were very physical and affectionate with each other, although in a nonsexual way. At Findhorn, to hug or touch another person is commonplace. It was natural for us to hug or walk arm in arm while in Scotland.

"We Norwegians do not touch each other in public. I'm nervous about either of you touching me, as much as I am about you and Daniel touching each other in front of anyone."

I assured her that we were guests in her home and in her country, and therefore we would be careful about any outward display of affection.

As Grete and I spoke of her fears, we noticed Daniel across the aisle talking to the woman next to him — she was in tears.

"What happened, if you don't mind my asking?" Daniel tenderly inquired.

"I've been in Scotland all week," she spoke with labored breath. "My father passed away. I've been living in Norway for years and never had as much time to spend with him as I wished I had. Now he's gone."

The plane's engines cast a dull roar in the background.

"This has been the worst week of my life."

She began to cry and her body shook. Daniel instinctively took her hands in his. It had a calming effect on her, and so she allowed him. After several minutes, he put one hand on her shoulder. They sat like that for over an hour. For the duration of the flight Grete and I tried to imagine what had happened. It then occurred to me that Daniel is a healer. He has an innate ability to sense and be compassionate to physical and emotional hardship. Through his gifted hands, he can heal pain. His body — any healer's body — is a by-product of the mind and spirit. Energy follows thought, and body follows consciousness. The distraught woman let him work freely in his healing, as she sensed he could help her. I was in awe.

In the terminal after we landed, Daniel told us what had happened. Not only had Daniel been given the last seat on the flight, he was also given a seat next to a woman who was in desperate need of his energy and healing abilities.

10

Entries/Entrées ***Visas*** *Departures/Sor*

332

The memories of our first day in Norway will forever be imprinted on my mind. Daniel had joined us only a day before, though it seemed we had been together always. I had met him briefly a week beforehand, and Grete just two days before. Yet the three of us found ourselves magically transported from Inverness, Scotland into Grete's living room in Bergen, Norway. Was it a dream? Instinctively we three knew our souls were at peace when we were together. We fitted naturally, like pieces of a puzzle. Even complete strangers sensed that our combined energies radiated differently from other people's. Merged together, we were guided in a direction we did not understand, but we absolutely could feel. We knew our purpose was genuine, but our question remained: What *was* our purpose?

Grete lives amidst a row of town homes that abut each other. We unloaded our belongings from the car and carried them towards her house. She was behind me as I searched for the correct door.

"Which number is yours?" I yelled back to Grete in confusion, because the doors all looked alike.

"332," she said laughing, "you know that!"

I chuckled when I realized I was truly at 332.

The comforts of Grete's home calmed us as we settled in. We had awakened extremely early that morning in Scotland, had traveled far, and were exhausted. A few hours remained before Grete's boys were to arrive from Denmark. She made hot water for us to sip. I lounged on the sofa in the living room, Daniel collapsed onto another sofa and

Grete sat in a chair nearby. My shoes and socks came off as we spoke quietly. Suddenly a cramp seized my left foot.

"Yow!" I screamed.

"What's wrong?" asked Daniel.

Impulsively I raised my knee to my chest and grabbed it. "I don't know. I haven't done anything to prompt any sort of muscle spasm."

"Here, give me your foot."

I stretched my leg towards him. He took it and began to massage it. "Just relax and breathe," he said calmly.

The pain was in the bottom of my left foot, about where the ball is. It was fortunate that Daniel was there. Trained in many types of massage, he is also a Reiki teacher. He learned Reiki, an ancient method of Japanese healing, when he lived in India. Reiki literally means universal life force. Daniel became a teacher, or master, through a multitude of initiations.

The pain subsided after he had massaged my foot for a little while. He placed my foot back on the sofa, and gently covered it with a blanket.

"I need to start to wash some laundry," Grete said as she left the room.

A moment after she left, Daniel stood. I remained where I was.

"I just remembered something," he said as he went into the laundry room with Grete.

Alone, I closed my eyes and attempted to relax on the sofa, but soon became agitated as I could somehow see Daniel and Grete. I saw not physically, because the laundry room was out of sight from the living room, but rather intuitively. It was clear to me they had closed the door and were kissing inside. Many emotions surged through me, but the strongest was jealousy. I was angry.

After a few minutes the laundry door opened. Grete came

out and went directly into the kitchen where I could actually see her. Daniel emerged a minute later, re-entered the living room and sat down. Grete served more hot water. We continued our previous conversation, but emotionally I was distressed because I knew what had just occurred. Our discussion was light, I couldn't focus on it.

"Aaaaagh!" I screamed suddenly.

My left foot was pierced by a fresh bolt of pain — in precisely the same spot it had been minutes before. The insult seemed a hundred times worse than the first time. It was of such an excruciating intensity I could hardly bear it. The spasm shot up my leg like liquid fire, and the strength of the shock thrust my entire body backwards. Abruptly I cried out and found myself in a completely horizontal position on the sofa.

"HELP!" I shrieked. "WHAT'S HAPPENING?"

The sheer agony dumbfounded me. I attempted to reach for my foot and felt a severe pang shoot up through my groin. It stabbed at my heart and then entered my head. When it twinged my throat I released a cry that I had never before heard come out of my mouth. I wondered where the sound came from. The torture of my shaking body was incomprehensible. Though my eyes were closed and full of tears, I sensed Daniel and Grete respond immediately. Grete put on music to help calm me and started to massage my feet, the source of my trial. Daniel flew to my chest and held me tightly around my heart.

"Breathe, breathe, breathe," he whispered as he embraced me, "breathe and let it all out."

"LET WHAT OUT?"

"All the pain and aches you have inside you."

I felt their unconditional love pour into me.

"Breathe, Tim, breathe, don't hold it in. Let this pain come all the way up and out of your body."

"I DON'T UNDERSTAND. TELL ME WHAT'S HAPPENING."

Daniel said quietly, "People pay thousands of dollars for therapy in hopes that something like this might happen to them, and you come to Norway for one hour and get it for free!"

I couldn't hear the humor in what he said. I could only feel the pain as it throbbed from the sole of my foot along the entire length of my body. My breathing was heavy and I shook as the convulsions pierced me. Groaning and aching, I continued to cry. I wanted to suppress the pain in my foot, because the intensity was too painful as it coursed through my body, but I listened to Daniel's words and let it come all the way out. The source was deep, buried in the bottom of my left foot. After more than twenty minutes my breath became more regulated and normal; somehow I sensed my waking nightmare had eased. Grete still tenderly massaged my feet, while Daniel continued his embrace.

"Daniel, I want to sit up and hold Grete too," I whispered to him in a barely audible voice.

We sat up so that they were on either side. In this way I was able to hold them both in my arms.

"I have no idea what just happened, but I do know I couldn't have made it through this ordeal without either of you."

There was a brief moment of silence.

"Do you want to talk about it now? Or do you want to wait until later?" Daniel asked.

A moment came and went. I knew I didn't need time.

"Now is OK."

"What do you think happened? What were your thoughts before the cramp began?"

Daniel and Grete were within inches of my face. At this close range it seemed even more difficult. My heart beat in trepidation, yet I had to tell them the truth.

"I saw both of you kissing in the laundry room."

They were puzzled because the door had been closed. Then they realized I had not seen with my physical eyes, but with my mind's eye. I glanced at Daniel and he just smiled. Grete's face, however, carried a look of guilt.

"I don't understand how I could see you two, but I did."

Grete spoke. "When Daniel and I were in there, I could see you too, but it wasn't your face I saw, it was my father's, and he demanded angrily of me 'Grete — what are you doing?'"

She paused.

"Tim," she said, "we're all together for a reason, but we know that, don't we? You know the left part of your body is the intuitive, female and emotional side, whereas the right part is the male — it's more practical and black and white. Your pain was buried in the bottom of your body, on the left side. You're confronting deeply emotional issues and so your suffering must have been difficult."

"It was."

I felt betrayed. It was not just because of Daniel; I realized there were other degrees of betrayal present in my life. My parents came into my thoughts. I remembered how there were times when I needed them, and they were not there. It didn't happen often, but there were a handful of events when I was growing up where I felt it important to have them present — from little league softball games to my high school graduation.

My dad had always kept a far distance from me until I became an adult. When I was a child I pretended that that was normal, that everything was OK. It wasn't. Years went by until I realized I was angry at my mom. She had stayed too long in an abusive marriage to a second husband. It was not a healthy environment for anyone to live in. Nearly two decades passed until she finally realized that she must get out. Her husband was too nice to me while at the same time he unleashed all his anger onto her. The abuse raged without end — it was the ultimate betrayal.

Who was to blame: Him, because he did it? Her, because she let him? Me, because I said nothing? And my own dad, where was he? As a child, I screamed from the inside, yet was too afraid to show anything on the outside. I had betrayed myself too.

These emotions were extremely difficult for me to acknowledge. I had buried them for most of my life because it was easier to suppress them than to confront them. As a child, I had handled my trauma in the best way I knew. However, I had reached a point where that denial was not functional for me any more. Suddenly my pain had surfaced — my soul made me face it so that I could move forward in my life.

Three hours had passed since our arrival in Norway, and I had already endured the most physically and emotionally traumatic experience of my life. My mind flashed back to Findhorn when Sandy had told me about metaphysics. I believed more than ever there was something to what she had shared with me. Perhaps Daniel and Grete did help trigger the response. The turmoil inside had been buried deep. It was necessary for them to help me alleviate and dispose of it. The source of what was buried deep inside, that ugly part of the past, departed forever.

The first night in Bergen I dreamed of a farm with a pig sty figuratively full of shit. A farmer arrived with a huge shovel, and proceeded to load all of the shit into a wheelbarrow to haul away.

I was in Norway to cleanse myself of a lifetime of accumulated garbage, and it was all being taken away. After only one day in Bergen I felt lightened of much of the baggage that invariably weighed me down. It was as though I had taken a vibrant deep breath of fresh air.

My astrologer had told me that in Norway I would find a strong energy. For me that energy represented the power to heal and be healed. I could never have understood the intensity of that healing force had I not allowed myself to share freely from the depths of my soul with my two friends.

On Tuesday night Grete's boys came home from Denmark. Normally she goes to a Reiki healing group on Tuesdays, but because she could not go that night, she invited Daniel and me to attend without her. We felt it ironic to be a part of a group Reiki healing session just hours after what had happened to me that afternoon with my foot. The leader, Kari, spoke English and therefore interpreted for us and to the others.

"Have either of you ever done or received Reiki healing?"

Daniel and I glanced at each other. I laughed as he smiled.

"I have received it, in fact just this afternoon . . . from him, and he's very good."

I pointed towards Daniel.

"Are you a trained Reiki master?"

"Yes, third degree," he shyly disclosed.

So began our evening as eight of us shared Reiki healing in peaceful surroundings in Norway. The experience was beautiful. We took turns lying on a table as the other seven people put their healing hands on our bodies. We felt rejuvenated when we left. It was only our first day, yet I knew I had accomplished so much. The day's experiences served to open Daniel and me to each other. He became more and more affectionate with me. A part of me became nervous when he touched me in front of total strangers. However, all our moods and emotions were completely open for us to question or discuss; there were no secrets or hidden agendas about anything. Never had I experienced such an honest relationship.

An expedition to the grocery store in the mall opened another door to our odyssey. Steffan and Stian, Grete's boys, were home, and so we all went together. However, after only a short time in the mall, we became emotionally disoriented from each other.

"I have to get out of here," I said.

"Me too," confirmed Daniel.

"The last few times I've been in this mall I've noticed how heavy I feel after only a few minutes," Grete commented. "Let's go."

Our depression continued even after we returned to the house. We decided a short hike into nature would ward off the negativity we seemed to have absorbed in the mall. A light mist hovered under the low cloud cover. The trees and bushes were saturated with heavy moisture, nevertheless we plodded on until we found a small clearing where we could rest. Crouching on the wet grass in our state of mental turmoil, we were silent for a long time as we listened to the sounds of the damp forest.

Finally Daniel spoke: "I don't know why I've come to Norway."

"I don't know how long I want to stay," I mumbled.

"I don't feel comfortable about sharing with either of you," Grete said. "I feel like retreating and going inside myself for a while."

We all had similar thoughts. We attempted to comprehend what had happened to us. It seemed we had hit a brick wall. Our meeting in Scotland, our travels to Norway — everything was finished. Suddenly a flash hit Daniel.

"Wait a minute! We haven't even been here 24 hours — and look what we've experienced in such a short period of time!"

Grete and I listened to him as he recapped only the last day in our lives. We then looked at each other in acknowledgement. We knew his observations were sound — the last 24 hours had been extraordinary for all three of us. Finally we smiled.

"You're right, my foot trauma was just yesterday afternoon."

"And actually I do want to share with you two," Grete confessed. "Please stay."

Joining hands and breathing deeply, we meditated for a short while despite the soggy grass. We inhaled the natural aromas of the Norwegian forest. Within only a few moments we felt our energies working together again. I felt we had been recharged — it hadn't taken long. We recognized we could not let ourselves be dragged down. When our jeans were completely soaked through, it was time to return home. We felt invigorated and refreshed.

Daniel and I were tense and overly conscientious regarding our physical contact with Grete or each other when the boys were home. Summer in Denmark had been fun with their father, but the boys were excited to be home with their mother. Steffan was eleven years old and Stian eight. Steffan proved to be always the shy one. His English was limited and so he was self-conscious about speaking in front of us. Stian, however, was extremely vivacious; he loved to impress Daniel and me with his knowledge of English. He tried so intently, sometimes we had to laugh.

"Mom . . . go . . . now . . . car," Stian announced one day when Grete was waiting for us outside.

"Takk!" we would respond to him, meaning thank you, the only word of Norwegian we knew.

We wondered what thoughts the boys had because their mom had brought home two men from her Scottish vacation. Perhaps they considered us a threat, or maybe new fathers for them. In actuality I don't believe they ever had any ill idea or fear of us. Grete, however, continued to be prudent in her protection of them. Daniel would cook dinners and I would do the dishes as we integrated into their home and family.

Daniel brewed chai for us, a tea he had learned to make in India by putting ginger, cinnamon, cardamom, anise, cloves, milk and honey in boiling water. The aroma makes it as wonderful to brew as it is to drink. The natural herbs soothe body and soul when sipped.

After our chai, Grete left the house to run a brief errand. There was some music I wanted to hear that I had bought at Daniel's suggestion, Mike Rowland's *The Fairy Ring*. I sat to write in my journal and Daniel sat nearby. Only a few moments after the music began, I thought I heard Daniel whimper. As I turned to look at him, I saw his eyes were full of tears. His hand was held out to me.

"Hold my hand," he whispered in a barely audible voice.

Daniel trembled as I held his hand tightly. He started to cry.

"I need you to hold me."

Moving to the sofa, I sat with him. He collapsed into my arms as he began to release all his emotions. He curled his entire body into my lap like a baby. Though competent to comfort him, I didn't understand why he was crying. The prospect that the boys might walk into the living room overwhelmed me, as they were in their room nearby. I didn't want Grete to be angry if they saw Daniel and me in an embrace. He bawled and shook with such intensity that for several minutes he could not utter a word. My heart stopped when I heard a noise in the next room — luckily it was Grete, who had returned. Daniel was knotted in my lap as I motioned for her to come over and help. She was puzzled as to what had happened, but then so was I. As we gave him our love, he slowly regained some strength. After several more minutes, his tears subsided and we were able to speak. *The Fairy Ring* continued to play in the background.

"Daniel, what happened?"

"This music reminded me of a time a few years ago that was very difficult for me."

Nervously I glanced at the door in hope that the boys would not walk in and encounter the three of us in a tight embrace. I was fearful as to what Grete thought of our situation, yet she was there with us, for Daniel.

"What happened a few years ago?" Grete asked gently.

"There were two things. First, my mom had been in the hospital with breast cancer for nearly three months. We didn't know if she would live or even be OK again. I was 21, and that was the first time in my life I had been without my mom. I didn't know if I'd ever see her again. Second, I had done some mild drugs at the same time, and knew I wanted to get off them and leave those friends behind. The trauma was incredible, but I did it. This CD of Mike Rowland is music I listened to a lot in that period, and I haven't heard it in a long time. I don't know why all this emotion came up now — but it did."

Grete and I gave our unspoken assurance with our smiles that we were there for him. We rocked him calmly in our arms. When Daniel had regained some emotional control of himself, Stian strode into the room — almost on cue. Oh no, I thought, now Grete will be angry. Stian, ever the show-off, impressed us again with his English.

"What's . . . goin' on?"

Grete motioned it was OK to come near. I was astonished. She explained to him in Norwegian what Daniel had just disclosed. Stian stared intently into Daniel's swollen eyes as his mom spoke. I could see in his tender young face that he could feel Daniel's pain. He reached to give Daniel a hug and then continued to look into his eyes with such endearing compassion. When Grete finished speaking, Stian slowly lifted his innocent little hand and placed it directly on Daniel's heart. It was a loving moment full of an eight-year-old's most spontaneous sincerity. Daniel's emotions were teetering on the edge, and so with Stian's action he again burst into tears and cried harder than before. Stian stood quietly and kept his hand on Daniel's heart until Daniel regained his composure. The most wondrous revelation came to me: this was but one of the reasons why the three of us had joined together — we needed to help heal one another of old wounds.

We all hugged each other. We found Steffan and put on some lively music. All five of us held hands and danced in the living room. We needed to lighten the heaviness of the morning, and it was a perfect exercise. Grete wept because her fear had diminished of what the boys would think of the three of us. They had magically become a part of our connected life force. She later confided to us that the boys began to call Daniel and me *healers* in Norwegian. It was OK to hug, to touch and be affectionate, because we were loving with them too.

Daniel's personal healing process integrated the boys with us. It represented a major step for Grete as she finally recognized and began to release many of her own fears. It was a ripple effect for her as this acceptance began with the boys and then quickly spread to her other family members and friends. She became free of her own fear. She was no longer distressed by other people's thoughts about what was contrary to normal society in Norway.

Grete had told us she had gone to a trance-channeler the year before.

"I feel that you two have a tremendous karmic bond," she said. "You can learn a lot about karma from a trance-channeler."

The thought excited and scared me at the same time.

"There's an American channeler in Bergen named William. He travels a lot, but if you two want, I'll try to find him for a session."

"Daniel, have you ever been to a channeler?" I asked.

"No."

"What do you say?"

"Let's go for it!"

"OK."

"Wait," Grete cautioned, "don't get too excited yet. My nephew and another friend have tried for more than a year to schedule a channeling with him — they've never been successful."

Her feeling was strong that we should try to meet with him. Daniel and I got on the same phone and listened as William's phone rang, our heads side by side.

"Hello this is William."

I was surprised he was home, astonished he answered.

"Hi, this is Tim."

"And this is Daniel," we declared nearly in unison.

"It was recommended that we call you for a channeling. We're in Norway on holiday after being in Scotland, and would like to know if it is possible to meet you."

There was a pause.

"When did you have in mind?"

"Maybe tomorrow?"

"Tomorrow? If there are two of you I'd prefer to do it on two different days because it's tiring to do."

We had a problem with transportation. He was quite a distance away and we knew it was only possible for us to go there once.

"Unfortunately we can't come on two different days," Daniel informed him. "Isn't there any other way . . . ?"

"OK, tomorrow at 1:00. I'll channel for one of you, take a break, and then channel for the other."

"Thank you very much!"

Grete was convinced it was important we see him. She knew it would help us in our understanding of ourselves as individuals, and of our relationship with each other.

The next day Grete dropped us off at William's home. My heart raced as we approached his front door. Daniel and I agreed I would be the first to proceed. He needed more time beforehand to meditate and become centered.

William answered the door and we exchanged brief formalities.

"Do you want to sit in on each other's sessions, or do you want to be private?"

"Private," Daniel said.

We were nervous.

"OK, each channeling will take about 1½ hours. Who's first?"

"He is," Daniel responded quickly.

We hugged, I entered, and Daniel relaxed outside on a deck chair.

William and I sat quietly for a few moments while he meditated in preparation. The room was quiet and I looked around while he sat with his eyes closed. In those few moments I felt skeptical. I had no wish to oblige him with any facts or clues as to who I was: not my age, what country I lived in, what sign I was — nothing. I considered it a test to see how good he was and if he really spiritually and intuitively could see into my past lives. Suddenly his eyes opened and he began.

"Your life's direction is to learn how to love unconditionally, and to let love come to you. Your problem in the past has always been that you're too mental and intellectual with everything and everyone. As a result you have always built a protective barrier around yourself so as not to let love come too close, lest it might hurt."

How true! He affirmed what many others have told me over the years.

"Earth is undergoing a purification process," he continued, "in order to shift into another dimension. It is cleansing all of the karma that we have brought in. It is also purging all of the negativity. Earth is triggering the process in itself, and therefore also in us. Those souls who resist the shift will fall apart and leave this earth. That's OK because they will reincarnate later. However, there is no fence to sit on. You have been fence-sitting, but you are now being provoked to go forward. It isn't a question of if you can, but if you will. You need to create a physical stimulus of energy to prompt your spiritual experience. This is the foundation of all that is happening to you."

"But why am I in Norway?"

"You frequently find yourself in diverse places all over the world. Initially you may think the purpose is to visit someone, take a course, or see a new city. That may be the how of where you go, but rarely is it the why. Different geographic places have specific karmic energies. Subconsciously you travel for and find this stimulation.

"Scotland is situated nearly in the center of the geographic third-eye energy center. You needed your third-eye stimulated, your intuitive abilities, and so you found yourself in such a place to support that process. The universe is using you as a human acupuncture to channel and anchor energy that will be instrumental for your development. As you receive this energy, you will find your mind opening.

"As for Norway, you must understand that Norwegians embody an incredibly fearful mass consciousness. It is a country full of self-denying souls. So many are afraid of their own feelings. They must trust and embrace compassion, but on the whole they are afraid to dare and go forward. You are here now to learn in the same way as they are. You must own the limitations you place on yourself all the time, and overcome your fear that you can't handle *self.* Your brakes are always on.

"You have a desire and need for intimacy on the deepest of all emotional levels. Your fear of losing control makes you unable to function. One of the greatest karmic lessons for all of us is that the more you fear something and avoid it, the more you will create it.

"Your higher self, your intuitive soul, is leading you. You must carry on and let it guide you as you advance and learn in order to ascend to the next level of your existence. Norway and western Sweden are the geographic world energy centers for the spiritual levels of all communication. They lie in the throat chakra. You are here at this time to help clear your ability as it relates to all forms of interaction and contact with people.

"In France in the 11th century there was a group of people called the Templars. They were the first people in a thousand years to begin publicly to question the church, and therefore the Pope. The Templars developed a business savvy that was looked down upon by the church. St. Augustine said, 'Business is in itself evil.' All economic activity had been severely repressed by the church for hundreds of years. The church taught that God was positive, but life on earth negative. Catholic Christianity tolerated little opposition as it dominated all philosophy in that day. Salvation was possible only from within the church and its teachings. Any other ideas were considered heretical.

"At the same time as the Templars, there was a group of nomadic people in southern France called the Cathars who had migrated from Bulgaria about 200 years before. They lived amongst the Templars and were therefore very influenced by them. By nature they were a loving and caring people — in fact Cathar means the pure ones. They preached salvation, not by way of Catholicism, but through personal achievement within themselves. They rejected the traditional teachings of hell, purgatory and the sacraments because of the material elements involved. Their own baptism was administered by the laying on of hands.

"Cathars were the first to give credence to free love. For example, they believed they should have the privilege of deciding whom they wanted to marry based on love. Until that period in time, the Pope, or the church, clearly determined who would marry whom — it never was a question of love. It was basically a denial of the sensual human — life was a continual struggle against the senses. The Cathars rejected this and many other sentiments. They loved and married as they felt.

"This was more than contrary to the church's teachings. The Pope felt undermined, and through the now infamous *Inquisition*, decreed all of these heretics be sought out and burned at the stake. Saint Augustine interpreted the scriptures as endorsing the use of force against heretics. It was quickly developed as common practice to seek out and charge any individual who seemed suspect. All Templars and Cathars were seen as a threat to both the ecclesiastical and social orders of the time.

"Tim, you were a Cathar. You could not conceive how, with the approval of religion, loving, caring people were burned to death because they believed in the privilege of choice. It was barbaric. You too were murdered by the Pope's men — this has left an impression on your soul that you have carried into all your incarnations. You desired to love, but were killed for it."

I don't remember if I breathed one breath as he spoke. I was overwhelmed — never could I have imagined this. Faintly I recalled the saga of the Templars and Cathars from history books. But me? A Cathar?

"You subsequently lived in central France as a monk," he continued. "You chose this life so you could hide behind the robe and the church in order to contemplate and learn without feeling human emotion. It was a sheltered and safe place to be. You had nothing to do but pray and interpret the written word. However, when you were in your mid-thirties, you met a younger monk and fell in love with him. He was innocent and beautiful. The love you discovered was instantaneous; you had finally found what you had been looking for. That young monk is waiting outside right now. That young monk is Daniel. You and Daniel have been together three times. You were also Celt warriors in Scotland, and young artists in Florence. All three times you were both men in love with each other."

The more William revealed, the lower I sank into the sofa. How was this possible? He didn't even know I lived in Florence now, in this lifetime!

"All three times you drew him into your heart. You had extraordinary relationships — especially as monks. Then after a time you panicked because it was too close, too emotionally intimate, and you eventually forced him away out of fear. This resulted time and time again in grave scars for you because you were apprehensive about loving, and always it was the deepest of sorrow for him.

"Your most powerful and creative incarnations have been in France and Italy, but especially Italy. You have lived there many times. Always you were great painters, musicians, writers and poets. Your creativity has always brought you into your full lovingness. When you express yourself creatively to people you are very powerful. It is frightening to the soul just how strong it is.

"Finally, about fifty years ago, you and Daniel met again," he continued. "This time, however, in very troubled circumstances. You were 12, and a German Jew at the outset of World War II. Daniel was a German 16-year-old, and was forced by his country to take part in the Jewish cleansings that Hitler commanded all German youth to participate in. Daniel was intensely against his country and this order by the state, but was fearful of what might happen to him or his family if he did not obey. You wandered onto the wrong street at the wrong time. Daniel and his group were on a rampage through the city. He was the first to see you. You actually came face to face with each other. He knew that when the others rounded the corner and spotted you they would beat you to a slow death. Because of the pressure on him, and out of compassion for you, he killed you there on the spot so you would not suffer at their hands in the ensuing onslaught. You knew your end was near, and made no attempt to run. Your soul let him do this atrocious deed for all the pain and suffering you had caused him. In this way, you two have come together again in this existence on equal ground."

In tears, I glanced out the window where I could see the back of Daniel's head as he sat on the deck. I told William we met in Scotland, I lived in Florence and Daniel lived in Berlin.

The smile on his face expressed no surprise.

"You have finally met again in Scotland. You are in Norway to clear the blocked passages of communication. Whether it takes a day, a week, or a lifetime, you two have much you need to share in your personal growth. You must learn to share love with each other unconditionally. This is why you have come together again."

"And Italy? Why do I live there now?"

"You have lived in Italy on numerous occasions. It feels good as your home now because it has been your home countless times. Your creative spirit is at its strongest in Italy. If you take full advantage of this ability, you will be successful with any artistic project you undertake. Please remember you have invariably sabotaged yourself in love. When you start expressing love, you inevitably detach yourself because of a foreboding that you might hurt the other person — or yourself. That is control. You must shake off that restraint, and simply let love be."

William rested while I left the house and joined Daniel outside. He stood as I neared him and we held each other tightly. Heavy with this new information, I felt too overwhelmed to speak. I didn't want to influence Daniel with anything before he went inside. It was necessary for me to remain in silence and begin the long process of assimilation.

After Daniel's channeling, he was in a stupor similar to mine. We both needed space and calm to reflect on what we had heard. Daniel's only comment immediately after his session was that perhaps he needed to come to Florence for a while. Later that day we compared notes. We realized William had communicated to each of us with unimaginable accuracy as to who we were as individuals. He had told Daniel things that could have been relevant only to Daniel. He had done the same with me.

The stories were of course parallel when he spoke of our shared lives. For Daniel, when World War II began, he enlisted to proceed to the front lines where he was promptly killed. He desired to be out, and got out. Daniel was born in Berlin in this lifetime. All through his school years he consistently had a difficult time when they would study World War II and the history of Berlin. He was always shocked at the atrocities and overwhelmed to the point where he could not — would not — read the text. William discerned he was born in Berlin because he had more lessons to learn there.

That night I dreamed I had taken an exam. I had arrived in the classroom to learn what grade I had received. After a search through the pile of other students' tests, I found mine. Bright red marks were scrawled all over it. The first two pages contained all the corrections. Suddenly I realized there was a page three and four. When I originally took the exam, I did not see those last two pages — I had not looked further than what I thought was there. I was nervous. Perhaps I had failed the entire course because of my negligence on this final exam. Quickly I turned to the first page to see if there was a final grade. There was none. Relieved, I glanced at the back two pages again to see what I had missed. A few of the questions were quite elementary while others were more complex. I thought if I had at least answered the simple questions I could have done better on the test.

The dream challenged me to look beyond my initial impression, and certainly further than what I believe I know. There is a multitude of possibilities open if I am intuitively aware. My life is an investigation of my soul's ability to accomplish my tasks at hand. I did not fail the exam; rather, it made me conscientious about being aware.

Friday morning was heralded by a bright Norwegian sun and clear blue skies. Grete announced the day would be perfect for the climb up the mountain behind her home. We all agreed. The mountain, Lovstakken, is one of seven that surround Bergen. An hour into the trek, our path wound around a pristine alpine lake that quietly nestled near the summit. It seemed to float almost mystically on the mountainside as it loomed over the surrounding landscape.

As we neared the crest, the trees cleared and the city of Bergen extended before us as if on an artist's canvas. The mountains, the fjords, the glistening city, even the sea in the background, seemed to stand attentively as if for our sole enjoyment. Breathless, I viewed the panorama below me.

"I have been here," I whispered to myself, "a week ago in Scotland."

Not one detail surprised me. Everything was accurately in its proper space. It was déjà vu.

"I can't put into words what I feel right now."

Daniel and Grete listened as I tried to share what I felt as I stood under the warm Scandinavian sun.

"This is exactly what I saw last week when I meditated. I didn't know then that Bergen was on the ocean. But I saw the city and the mountains and the sea all at the same time. And now here I am. I'm actually looking at the reality of the parallel reality that Britt told me about!"

It was perfect. The air I breathed was peaceful and clean. How could I have been here in my mind? How could I have intuitively seen a week ago what I never could have physically imagined a week ago? In the quiet of August, we felt only a soft wind under the blue skies on top of Lovstakken.

"Do you two know what my angel card was at Findhorn?" Grete asked.

"No."

"It was Surrender."

"And what did you learn from that?" questioned Daniel.

"Actually I think I'm just now beginning to learn."

We listened respectfully.

"Daniel, the first two days after I met you I had romantic feelings for you," she said. "I've released those feelings because I know they aren't realistic. I've surrendered them and I feel much better."

"Thank you for sharing that," he responded.

We parted for an hour to meditate on our own. I found a grassy site and as I settled comfortably I recognized that even my seat was the same as I had envisioned when I meditated at Findhorn. I believed I would have the next part of my adventure roll across the screen of my mind as I sat with my eyes closed on the peak of Lovstakken — simple guidance for what to do next.

My meditation lasted perhaps an hour. Desperately I searched for one more clear image to find direction. Nothing. What had happened? The meditation was pleasant, but failed to meet my personal expectations. Standing, I stretched in the warm sun, and went to join Daniel and Grete. They knew I was in great anticipation. Daniel too was searching for an indication of what he needed to do.

"How are you?" they inquired as I neared them.

"Fine. I'm really thirsty."

We drank some refreshing water we had brought with us.

"Nothing came to me," I finally confessed. "I don't understand, I was sure my coming to this mountain would direct me towards what will be my next step. I don't know what to do. How were your meditations?"

"Mine was nice, very peaceful," said Grete. "The only idea that came to my mind was that maybe you two need to call William. He was so open and receptive about seeing you, maybe he has more to tell you."

"And your meditation, Daniel?"

"Mine was good too, but pretty normal for me," Daniel related. "It felt great to sit here under the sun, the warmth was comforting, but I didn't get any sense of what to do next. I'm confused because tomorrow is the day I was to return to Berlin from London. I feel pressured by Tessa to go home. I don't know what to do."

Before, direction had seemed to come our way effortlessly. I had great expectations about meditating on the mountain because I had seen it a week before. Daniel did not know when to leave Norway. Neither did I, but I didn't feel the pressure he felt to return home. The time had come for us to hike down; the boys would be waiting for us at the house. We literally ran down the mountain like deer. It was invigorating to breathe and fill our lungs with the pure air. The exercise balanced the needs of our bodies.

The boys greeted us with the news that someone had telephoned us. We wondered who it could be because no one knew where we were.

"Who called for us?" I quizzed Stian.

"Someone . . . ask . . . for . . . you and Daniel . . . in . . . English," Stian proudly responded. "He . . . call back."

"It was William," Grete quickly discerned, "he must have called for you. Did you give him this number?"

"No."

"How could he know you were here? He doesn't know my number," she wondered aloud. "Did he ask you my last name when you saw him?"

"No."

We never did understand how he found us.

"I still have his number, let's call him now," I urged Daniel.

It was indeed William who had called earlier. He had

wanted to see if Daniel and I could have lunch with him on Sunday. We agreed immediately, and set a place to meet in downtown Bergen on Sunday afternoon.

"I suppose that's a sign that I won't go home tomorrow," Daniel declared laughing.

"Guess so," I agreed. "Maybe we should have listened more attentively to Grete on the mountain. She was sure William had something more to tell us."

We learned a valuable lesson that day: when we are in the flow and centered, we will always be led by our soul. However, we cannot anticipate when, where, how and why this direction will come to us. If we try too hard to figure it out mentally, it will only tease us and appear from another unexpected angle. We just need to be open and patient, and trust that guidance will come.

Saturday morning as I awakened, focusing on the first flickering moments of consciousness, an image of Daniel and myself came to mind. We were away from Grete and the boys. It was a type of bed-and-breakfast cabin somewhere on the coast, with the sea in the background. The perception was fleeting and I realized I had just experienced another parallel reality. Daniel agreed it sounded good when I shared my idea with him. We talked and decided Monday would be a good day to leave. We mentioned to Grete our plan to find a secluded place for relaxation for two or three days. She liked the idea too.

Our newly-formed Norwegian family — Grete, Steffan, Stian, Daniel and I — decided to spend the day in downtown Bergen. We enjoyed an outdoor lunch under the warm sun at a wharf-side restaurant. The fjords with their magical towering cliffs meander in and out between the high rises of the city, dwarfing Bergen with their grandeur. It is a dramatic and impressive city and the views are spectacular from every angle.

Grete and the boys left us later in the afternoon to run errands. Daniel and I slowly wandered through the streets, taking in the city's many sights. We stumbled on an Indian restaurant for our dinner.

During our meal, Daniel noticed fear in my eyes. "What's wrong?" he inquired.

We knew each other too well by now to hide anything.

"I'm thinking about your coming to Florence. I'm uneasy about having you come so near into my life. My mind thinks a relationship with you would be too hard: you live in Berlin, you are ten years younger — and you have a girlfriend! My heart wants to love, but my reasoning mind says it will be too hard."

"At least you are aware of it," he said soothingly. "In this way you can fight and overcome the negative parts of the ego and just let the heart sing."

"Easy for you to say."

"Actually it's not!"

We each intuitively always stepped in with strength when the other needed it. In this way we helped teach each other and ourselves at the same time.

Our dinner conversation eventually lightened. We spoke of Italy, and of what Berlin was like for him before and after the wall came down. We arrived very late at Grete's home. She had waited up for us because she had exciting news to share.

"So much has happened in only a few hours! I had two calls. The first was from Jan-Helge and Britt. They are in London."

"Already?"

"Yes. Tim, I told them what happened with your foot, and Britt suggested that perhaps Daniel had inflicted the pain in another lifetime. She explained that he had the ability to help heal now the hurt he had caused at another time."

"Wow," we both responded.

"And then an hour ago," she continued, "the phone rang again. It was a lady by the name of Kavito who is a friend of Kari's. I have met her once. She and her husband live two hours south of here on an island called Reksteren. She telephoned because she heard I had two foreigners staying with me, and she thought it might be agreeable if you two could go and spend some time at their place on their remote island. She and her husband are leaving for a holiday — their place is yours if you want it."

"I don't believe it," Daniel muttered.

"Neither do I," I agreed.

It had happened again! All we needed to do was imagine something, and it materialized!

"Daniel, obviously this means we must go to their island."

"Let's call her now."

"It's too late tonight," said Grete. "We'll call her first thing in the morning."

"Why did she call us?" I wondered. "What prompted her?"

"I have no idea, she didn't say," Grete answered as she attempted an explanation. "I've only met her once, but you two announced this morning you wanted to leave for a few days. When she called out of the blue, I just felt it was right!"

"Wait," Daniel broke in, as he struggled to understand, "this woman who you don't really know, happens to call to inquire if your two house guests, who are complete strangers to her, might possibly be looking for a cabin to stay in on a remote island for a few days?"

We all burst out in laughter.

"Yes!"

"We must be living in a fantasy. None of these coincidences seem to be real!" Daniel asserted.

"Did she say when we can go?" I questioned.

"Yes," Grete laughed again, "she mentioned Monday, just the day you two thought you might want to go."

"Grete, you must be making this up," I stated in disbelief, yet I knew she spoke the truth.

We laughed and laughed. Our path was further cleared as we continued our journey. The next morning we called Kavito.

"Hi, this is Daniel."

"And this is Tim."

Again we shared the phone receiver.

"Hi! Are you two interested in coming to our cabin for a few days?" Kavito asked.

"Yes, of course we are, we would love to!"

Our smiles were so broad, nothing could have brought us down.

"Is tomorrow all right? There's a ferry that leaves Bergen at 11:00 in the morning. It's a breathtaking journey through the fjords by boat. You'll be here by 2:00, and I will meet you at the dock. Is that OK?"

"It's perfect," responded Daniel, "but just a moment, I have a question. Why did you call us?"

"I don't know. I heard Grete had two friends here. Our place is beautiful and we need someone to feed the dogs and chickens while we are away. I simply felt you might be open to coming out here."

"That's all I wanted to hear. We'll be on the ferry at 11:00 tomorrow!" Daniel affirmed.

"Her voice sounded so calm over the phone," he acknowledged after he hung up. "It was good to talk to her. I know it's right that we go!"

"I'm with you," I said. "Why do these miracles keep happening to us?"

"You always try to figure out the reasons," Daniel answered bravely. "We don't always know the why behind everything. We know this is right, so let's just go with it!"

William fascinated us with his lunchtime conversation. We had many questions to ask, and as always the time flew quickly.

"How were we able to get a channeling with you when we had called only the day before," Daniel queried.

He smiled. "Actually, I stopped doing channelings about a year ago. I write, lecture, and travel too much. It keeps me very busy. However, when you two called me, there was no doubt in my mind that I would meet with you. I can't explain it. — I simply felt it was necessary."

"So what is our mutual purpose, having come into each other's lives?" I asked.

William spoke like a sage: "Daniel is a mirror of the inner child you never allowed yourself to be. And you are a mirror of stability that Daniel has never known. You two are two sides of the same coin."

As William spoke, Daniel scribbled some thoughts on the back of a postcard:

My life is really flying right now. I hope I continue to have the faith to stay on. The things I am perceiving now seem so confusing. Sometimes fear pops up all over the place, but I am less and less deterred/swayed by it. I still try to think what's ahead, to plan to hold on, to follow/allow my feelings.

After he wrote, he paused and looked William square in the eye.

"So why are we in Norway?" Daniel challenged.

"You're both in Norway to learn how to own your own feelings, and follow your own truth."

William's answers were direct, and after some consideration we realized we were not surprised by them. However, one of his comments did startle me.

"Tim, Daniel is the only soul that has ever broken through the emotional safety barrier with which you have always surrounded yourself."

On our last night at Grete's, Daniel dreamed of an ocean that he could not see through to the bottom. Grete and I swam freely, but he was afraid of sharks if he went into the wrong part. After a time Grete and I had put away our towels and clothes that were no longer important to us. He ran after us because he was afraid to put his valuables away.

For me, water represents our feelings. Daniel still felt fearful about venturing too far into his emotions. He was reluctant to put away the things that he had always felt were important to him up to that point in his life. The sharks were making him face old obstacles as he developed a relationship with me that was still too unknown to him.

I dreamed I prepared to move into a round house. Everything was round and smooth. There were many things in the kitchen and bathroom that would need renovating before I moved in.

The round house was unity and totality. I foresaw the work I had yet to do before I could achieve that state of wholeness. The odyssey continued.

10

1100 Ducks

The ferry ride through the fjords of Norway was spectacular. The warm summer sun highlighted the mountain peaks from above, and reflected down into the icy blue water below. Chalet-style homes dotted the meadows and mountainsides with cheery flowers hanging from their window boxes. The steeply-pitched roofs reminded me that winter descends like a tempest in this part of the world. I attempted to visualize the landscape and homes blanketed in white snow. The Scandinavian sky provided a dramatic backdrop that day as the brilliant blue met the tops of the fjords like something on an artist's canvas. It seemed a fairy-tale, so peaceful in its tranquillity. It was warm enough to stand outside on the deck of the ferry. The brisk wind clipped by as our boat navigated the water passages. We held our faces towards the sun and drew in the life energy we felt coming from its warm rays. Standing side by side we gazed dreamily out over the watery landscape. It was hypnotic to watch the cobalt blue water as it slipped quickly underneath the hull of the speeding boat. It was one of those rare and beautiful moments when I realized that all is well and good within me. Daniel put his arm around me affectionately. The windows of the captain's bridge were directly above and behind us.

"Are you trying to rile the captain and his crew by holding me in their full view?"

"Yeah, so what will they do, throw us overboard?" he joked.

The trip through the fjords took about three hours. On the way I thought of the map that had guided me to this place. I was mesmerized by our adventure of love and healing that propelled me to embrace more of what life meant.

Kavito had said she would pick us up at the dock on the island. Not many people or cars disembarked at our stop at Reksteren. We marched off the boat and attempted to imagine what she looked like. Within a minute the ferry blew its horn as it anxiously announced its departure. We looked for anyone who might be looking for us. The few cars and people that were there dispersed quickly and left us alone at the dock. We laughed at ourselves in diversion. We were completely alone on a ferry dock on an island in the Norwegian Archipelago without direction and without a ride. At least the sun felt good on our shoulders.

Suddenly we heard a loud engine as a truck barreled down the hill to the dock. It was a big blue four-wheel drive, with a pretty blonde woman at the wheel. She seemed out of place in such a vehicle, but it was obvious Kavito loved it.

"You Daniel and Tim?" she shouted out the window as she pulled up to the only two people who stood on the dock.

"Hey Kavito!"

We greeted her in unison and tossed our luggage into the back, leaping into the high truck for the brief ride to her cabin. Her driveway was through a locked gate and up about a mile of steep and weather-worn rutted dirt roads. We realized this truck was the only kind of vehicle to have if one lived in such a remote and isolated place. It was almost necessary to wear a seat belt on the drive between her gate and the house. The road was so rough our heads kept hitting the ceiling with every bump and dip we drove over.

Their cabin nestled between two sheer rocky mountain ridges that were so close they seemed to touch each other. They were covered with vibrant Norwegian firs that seemed to grow out of every crack and crevice. As a result, the views were literally breath-taking. Their cabin was painted a rich cranberry red, with an autumn gold trim. The contrast was beautiful against the mountains and sky. The sea lay in the background. It was a picture postcard setting. We recognized how privileged we were to enjoy this rare place of pristine natural beauty. Behind their home was a miniature replica of their cabin, painted in the same fashion. It was a house for roosters and chickens. They had no sewage system, so the toilet was behind and beyond the main cabin. I couldn't imagine what it must be like to live there in the winter and always need to go outside to use the toilet. It was a rustic but beautiful existence. Beyond their cabin were several other bird enclosures.

"It's a duck farm," Kavito explained as we unloaded our belongings from the truck.

We chuckled to ourselves. Neither of us had ever been on a duck farm.

"Before we go on holiday, we must do our last round-up of the year," she told us. "Would you two like to help us corral all the ducks so they can be taken away? In a few hours some of our neighbors on the island will come to help as well."

"Sure," we said trustingly, without any idea of what we were committing ourselves to, much less how to corral ducks. I laughed to myself as I tried to imagine a stampede of ducks quacking and honking.

From where we stood we could see down a hill into a fenced-in enclosure, with perhaps two dozen geese and ducks inside.

"How many do you have?" Daniel inquired casually.

"Eleven hundred."

"Eleven hundred ducks!"

We roared with laughter. Our odyssey continued to astonish us as we turned corners we never could have foreseen or prepared for.

Daniel confided to me: "We wanted a holiday break at a cabin. We got it. We just didn't imagine we'd have to work once we got here!"

Who would have known? Kavito's husband and five of their neighbors prepared for the grand event. Kavito loaned Daniel and me overalls to wear, as she admitted that we would become very dirty — and we hadn't packed duck-corralling clothes for our adventure. A large semi somehow made it up the steep and treacherous dirt drive, and we unloaded over two hundred duck crates from it. They explained that they went through this process three times a year, and tonight was our lucky night because we could help!

The ducks lived in some woods that were down behind the main cabin. They are fattened with high-protein food and eat so much they cannot fly. Many are barely able to walk. As ducks go, they are beautiful with snowy white feathers and extremely long necks. We were told if we needed to we could actually pick them up by the neck, as it would not hurt them. Ducks are certainly not the cleverest of creatures, so when we began the round-up with whistles and screams to herd them toward the corral, many froze with fear.

"I can't believe I'm abetting a duck slaughter!" my vegetarian friend Daniel commented.

"Look at us!" I responded with a chuckle. "What are we doing on an island in Norway rounding up ducks?"

We knew we had to try to rationalize what we were doing because the reality of the experience was so incomprehensible. We found we did have to pick up and carry some of the ducks. Many of them stuck their heads in the fence in hopes we would not see their fat bodies sticking out behind them. After we got them into the tight corral, we had to load them — five per crate. That's when the job got dirty! They screeched and honked and waddled and cried out in fear as we placed them individually into their crates for transportation. After they were all loaded, they became eerily quiet as they were driven away to their destiny. What an experience!

At the celebration dinner afterwards, Kavito interpreted for us as most of the island neighbors did not speak English. They were a quiet but hard-working people who lived full time on the island. Daniel and I were humbled by the opportunity to share with these islanders, many of whom have little contact with the outside world. We enjoyed a warm and hospitable old-style Norwegian potluck dinner.

With eleven hundred ducks now gone, we knew at least we would not have to feed as many birds. However, there were plenty of other animals. They had a collection of dogs, as well as chickens and roosters. They showed us how to care for their pets, and departed early the next morning for a long overdue vacation in France.

We awakened to the sound of the dogs howling eerily. They intuitively sensed their owners had left. Their howls echoed back and forth between the rocky mountain sides. The early morning mist hung as if suspended by wires between the steep slopes that enclosed us in our own little canyon. We simultaneously commented that it felt a bit like Transylvania! We slept in the guest quarters above a garage and noticed an odd odor in the air. A steep ladder led to our room. Near the top of the ladder we found several boxes that seemed to be the source of a particular smell neither of us had ever experienced before. Further exploration revealed that they were full of hundreds of dried pigs' ears and tails! They were as horrible to see as they were to smell.

Our adventure held infinite surprises.

Behind the main cabin was a lovely grassy area. A wooden deck connected the cabin to the grass and to some oversized natural boulders that jutted out of the landscape. The morning sun rose behind us in this paradisical setting while we enjoyed our morning breakfast and tea. We hadn't a care in the world.

Suddenly, clouds surrounded the island, and a rain began that offered to cleanse and heal at the same time. It was a light, summer, misty rain, and in that setting, tucked between the mountain sides, with the clouds low over the horizon, it seemed mystical. We almost expected a white unicorn to gallop by the cabin windows. Once in a while the dogs would begin to howl in their loneliness. We were lost and light-years distant from any hint of civilization.

Daniel gave me a wonderful massage. The word *peace* echoed continually through my being as his hands worked. When he had finished, we shared our Indian chai, then started a discussion about ourselves that was to last two days. It was so healthy to be learning how to confront all our feelings directly and honestly, including hurts and misunderstandings.

"Daniel, do you realize we have been together twenty-four hours a day for the past ten days, and we aren't the least bit tired of each other?"

"Yeah, a woman in India told me there is only one soul in the world that is perfectly compatible with my own. I wonder if you are it?"

"I don't know if there is only one other soul for each of us, but we do have harmony."

If there was anything we had not talked about until that point on the island, we shared it then. We dived into the deepest recesses of all our secrets. Taking turns, we told of incidents from our lives that few if any people knew about.

We challenged each other and revealed ourselves from the depths of our souls.

"What is your greatest fear?" I asked.

"My greatest fear?"

"Yes."

Daniel chuckled as he thought. "Hmmm . . . Probably myself."

"Really? Sometimes I feel the same."

"It's amazing. Often when I'm ready to step forward with something, my fear soars so high that I stop. But this trip has been incredible for me, because I didn't let my fear rise too high — well sometimes I did, but I have learned how to step through it instead of letting it block me."

"Daniel, everything has flowed for us without a single problem. We have never had any idea what we would do from one day to the next — look at the last ten days of our lives!"

"It was effortless, every single thing we did — totally effortless."

We sat facing each other on a small sofa, the only sofa in the cabin. It was as if both our minds went into high-speed reverse, reflecting back on all our shared experiences since we had met. The August rain had stranded us inside.

"Do you think we can live like this forever, even when we get back into the real world?" I asked.

"Oh, that real world thing. It's possible, but I think it is a lot harder. We've been on vacation, so we haven't had to deal with the day-to-day stress that smacks us in the face in that real world."

"I think we've been shown how to live while we're here," I stated, "because this environment is easier to learn in. Now it's our job to make it work in our regular lives."

"Yeah. You know, we have carried each other through many lessons."

"Daniel, that means we have faith in ourselves and in each other."

"It's incredible because usually my fear limits me so much. I know I could never have had any of these opportunities if I had let my fear — my ego — get in my way."

"When we let our energies be channeled by fear, instead of light, our flow stops completely."

"Aha, it's all back to light, isn't it?"

"Seems to be."

"So fear must be our greatest weakness."

"That's the feeling I'm getting from what we have learned."

I felt so good as I realized we had helped each other look deep inside ourselves.

"You know that when we are in the flow like this, we are in control. This is how we create our own reality. Our souls will never lead us wrong . . ."

"As long as we listen!" I finished for him.

"So our life is what we make of it, not what our society has molded for us — or what we carelessly let happen. We were, we are, completely in charge of our own destinies."

"Bingo."

We spoke with profound intensity as we helped each other understand all that had happened.

"Daniel, take one example of how our souls guided us."

"Which one?"

"Any. How we met at the Park for example."

"That's a good one."

"I remember you told me a messenger had come to tell you that you must leave the bed and breakfast."

"Yeah, it wasn't the owner, it was a messenger."

"Exactly, it was a messenger, a guide, an angel — whatever — telling you it was time to move forward."

"Tim, that messenger guided me. And yeah, I remember using the word messenger."

"Who was that messenger? Your guardian angel? The voice of your soul? Your light?"

We laughed.

"So you came to stay with us," I continued. "But I wouldn't have been in the camper at the Park if there had been a bed at Newbold House."

"I thought about that."

"And you probably wouldn't have met the Norwegians if it wasn't for me."

"I know."

"And Grete and I almost took the boat across from Scotland. If we had, we would have left before you and I actually ever met at the Park. We went by plane because that is what I saw in my meditation."

"And you had to wait for me!"

"That's right."

And now here we are on a duck farm on an island in Norway in someone's cabin who doesn't know us."

"Unbelievable, I know."

"It's all part of the flow!"

"So, Daniel, we are guided if we let ourselves be — and we did."

"The last ten days have not been a series of accidents."

"No, our three souls led us all toward each other because we had work to do with and for each other."

For me, our time together represented a major leap forward in my own maturity. It was the first time for both of us that we had been so naturally intimate with another person without consummating our relationship. Though our attraction was certainly also physical, it proved necessary first for our souls to evolve spiritually together. We intuitively understood that as we created this strong base, our relationship would be everlasting — as apparently it had already been. And then, from the insight that would come from the depths of our souls regarding our future, we would step forward onto the next level of our lives together. Our unconditional love for each other gave us incredible strength. As a result I learned to love another's inner being first, instead of just the outer personality.

We discussed our future together, and what direction our relationship would take after our departure. Daniel determined he would come to Italy to spend time with me. We agreed never to harbor secrets and vowed always to continue a relationship of pure honesty. The unconditional love we felt had not just sprung up in the past few weeks; rather we had been developing it over many lifetimes. As William said, we simply came back together where we left off the last time.

"Daniel, this has been the most exhausting and emotional vacation I've ever had. I have worked harder, learned more, cried more, cleaned out more, and dug deeper into the very core of who I am than I have ever done in my life. My holidays have never been like this before — I thought I was going to have a rest!"

"There doesn't seem to be much time to rest any more. Everything seems to be going faster and faster. There is so much to do. I know I have to make some major changes in my life when I go home."

"Can you make those changes?"

"Yes. I've learned in the last few weeks that I have no choice but to make changes. I normally get so afraid, but I feel strong now."

"You know, we have a balance with each other that I've never felt with anyone else."

"Yeah, what is it William said? Two sides of the same

coin?"

Our time in Norway was nearly over. Destined to cross paths again, our souls had rejoined each other. I had learned how to love Daniel with my heart — not my ego. It felt great.

We had told Kavito before her departure that we wanted about three days at her cabin. She informed us that another friend was to arrive on the third day, which, if we desired, would allow us the freedom to leave. Magically on the third day, we both felt it time to go. The synchronicity once again was flawless. We prepared our bags and hiked the long way down the rocky drive and then to the dock to catch the ferry to Bergen. The boat trip was bittersweet. We were excited to go on to the next step in our lives, but also sad to leave what had been a most idyllic adventure.

On the way back to Bergen, Daniel drifted off to sleep and dreamt of the cabin on the island. He stood at the kitchen door, and I stood atop a large boulder a little ways away. There was a heavy cable drawn between the rock I stood on and the cabin. I had just swung out to the rock on the cable using a bar, like in a circus, and sent the bar back to him so he could join me. I held the cable taut and strong so he could come without fear of it breaking or swinging. He stood at the kitchen door, ready but still hesitant to come to the rock.

When Daniel awakened he hugged me warmly. He confided what he had dreamt, and told me he felt he could truly rely on and trust in me.

Back at Grete's, we called the airport. There was an early flight to Copenhagen the next day. We knew we both needed to connect there with flights to our individual homes.

The time to leave was approaching. Our reunion with Grete, Steffan and Stian was wonderful. It seemed an eternity since we had seen each other, yet only three days had passed. Grete had prepared a dinner of fresh Norwegian salmon for our final meal. She doesn't like to cook, but we could feel the love she had put into the preparation of it. It was incredibly good, and as we ate she shared some remarkable news.

"One of my neighbors approached me and wanted to know of my experience at Findhorn," she said. "I don't know how they understood what kind of place it was. Suddenly my heart was open — I wasn't afraid, and I shared with them. I was shocked at myself because I talked about it openly. They had noticed a difference in me. When they had seen you two around, they didn't feel threatened by you in the way I thought they might."

"See, Norway isn't so bad after all," I teased.

We all laughed. Grete had transformed dramatically in only ten days. Her fears were erased. Steffan and Stian continued to call us healers.

"The first thing we did was to help heal each other," Grete said. "It began with Tim's foot on the first day, and then with Daniel's music experience with his mom. That led to Steffan and Stian coming into our extended family, which in turn led me into a circle of people I had been afraid to share with."

Daniel and I could see by the glow on her face that she felt as good inside as she did out.

"That's true," I added, "and because of those healing experiences, we learned how to provide and give unconditional love and support. We're strong now and I feel we are ready to return to our lives we left behind a few weeks ago."

"And for Tim and me," Daniel related, "we needed to get to know each other here in this setting for whatever may come of our relationship in the future."

"We were brought together to help each other in our continuing development," Grete declared. "We can't help heal anyone else until we ourselves are whole."

"Our angels, or guides, continually interacted with us whether we recognized their presence or not," added Daniel. "They taught us to radiate love from within."

"You know, you two were more evolved in spiritual matters than I was before we met in Scotland," I said. "Thank you for what you have taught me. The three of us being together while we've been here in Norway has moved me in ways I had never imagined. I have found a strength within myself that was yearning to be used and set free. I'm a completely different person."

Daniel gazed out the window before he spoke again. "It doesn't matter where you come from, or where you are. If you have trust and faith in yourself — then you can move mountains! Everything is possible. In the last fifteen days, we have never asked or inquired about anything. All our experiences have happened as we trusted in the moment."

"The unusual, the unknown, the non-conventional — I've learned to accept it all," I said.

"True. We have also learned how to combine our soul-energies into our routine lives," Grete observed. "They go together easily, though I did not think they could for me. I, maybe I need to say we, created our own lessons of reality. Findhorn opened us, and then we took a quantum leap forward."

As we prepared to leave, I became more reflective. "You know, we each have a powerful energy that can change the course of humanity — that sounds big, I know. What we three did was great and it carried us into wonderful experiences. But can you imagine if our number wasn't three, but three hundred, three thousand, or three million? If three million people listened to the voices of their hearts and souls

— what would happen to humankind?"

"Wow!"

"It's humbling to think about," I continued. "Our power is within when we create our own reality. So, as we align ourselves, our energies will work together. Remember how when we consciously stayed centered and lived and believed in the moment — not in yesterday or in tomorrow — how the doors in front of us always opened literally just before we reached for the handle?"

We all laughed. It was so true.

"It's not just us," Grete said, "people everywhere are seeking to transform and improve their lives. I don't think this change is coming from the external world — I feel it's coming from within ourselves. An evolution is taking place. As people, we all have our own lessons to accomplish and healings to complete. That is the journey."

Our experiences in Scotland and Norway have forever bound the three of us. We came together not simply by a fluke of luck, but rather because of a divine intervention of fate in our lives. We are strikingly stronger and more courageous today than we were before. Collectively we also realize our responsibilities are intensified as we carry on with our journey. Our subconscious acceptance to be healed has led us to develop further our abilities to heal. It is with this knowledge and energy that we go out into the world to continue our lives' tasks.

On our last morning, Grete, Daniel and I had our final tune-out. We asked for and gave ourselves strength to go forward as we prepared to leave each other. We felt good knowing we had each resolved many of our own inner conflicts. Our new power was exhilarating.

Daniel and I were able to board the same flight to Copenhagen. Our adventure was fast coming to a close. Daniel was nervous because he knew within a few hours he would be with his family and Tessa. He had many new truths to share with all of them because of his experiences in Scotland and Norway. He knew he had many changes to make in his life as a result of his opening and newly expanded conscious awareness.

I felt excited to return home to my own environment. I knew I would never view the world in quite the same way again. It was as if I had slowly learned to focus my eyes — the trees were greener, the sky was bluer, and people were more real.

In Copenhagen airport we sat in what we later realized was the helicopter waiting lounge. It was full of conservatively-dressed businessmen. Daniel and I held hands and closed our eyes as we felt our joined energies circulate through our bodies. I knew all the men must have been watching, but I didn't care. Soon we heard the page for Daniel's flight to Berlin. He slowly leaned forward and kissed me. Our Norwegian odyssey was over, but our journey was just beginning.

10

Afterwords

The final words for *Journey* were written nine months after our actual journey. I hadn't understood the real reason behind my foot trauma when it happened. And in fact, when I wrote about it, I wondered how to describe it, because I truly had no explanation. As my soul guided me in the writing, I discovered exactly what my past issues had been with betrayal. When I realized my own personal awakening had taken place nine months after the fact, I felt that period of time was very appropriate. It was as though the thought of betrayal had been conceived in August in Norway, and the actual birthing had happened nine months later in April in Italy. I hadn't been ready to accept and deal with those issues at the time. My process was difficult to come through when I realized this — however it has been very fulfilling.

Daniel came to Florence for the month of October in 1995. Our time together was incredible, even though when he came I had still felt unsure about being with him. Meeting him had led me down many unknown paths, and so I decided to allow him into my life as these paths had always turned out to be good ones. Every day was a new adventure for us and I realized he was a pattern-breaker for me. He was also my inner child. He rearranged my eating, my sleeping, my home, my life — and I let him. It was wonderful, and I gave myself a gift of freedom that I had never had before. We laughed together, thought together, and taught each other patience and tolerance. I learned to live for the now, not for what had been, or what could be.

October 1996 — *Journey* is nearly ready to go to print. I have just returned from Berlin where I attended the wedding ritual of Daniel and Tessa. With only a few close friends and family present, it was an uncommonly beautiful celebration of love. My feelings were warm and compassionate as I saw and felt the love they share. Grete is very busy raising her two beautiful sons in Norway. Jan-Helge and Britt have been traversing the globe, and the past year has found them in Egypt, India, America and Mexico. My destiny has brought me together with Anand, who has become my companion.We are fondly reflecting on our own travels through India just this past summer, where we spent a month exploring our love for the land, for the people, and for each other.

The journey continues.

Introducing Findhorn Press

Findhorn Press is the publishing business of the Findhorn Community which has grown around the Findhorn Foundation, co-founded in 1962 by Peter and Eileen Caddy and Dorothy Maclean. The first books originated from the early interest in Eileen's guidance over 20 years ago and Findhorn Press now publishes not only Eileen Caddy's books of guidance and inspirational material, but also many others. It has also forged links with a number of like-minded authors and organisations.

For further information about the Findhorn Community and how to participate in its programmes, please write to:

The Accommodation Secretary
Findhorn Foundation
Cluny Hill College
Forres IV36 0RD
Scotland
Tel. +44 (0)1309 673655 Fax +44 (0)1309 673113
e-mail: reception@findhorn.org
url: http://www.gaia.org/findhorn/index.html/

For a complete catalogue or more information about Findhorn Press products, please contact:

Findhorn Press
The Park, Findhorn, Forres IV36 0TZ, Scotland
Tel. +44 (0)1309 690582 Fax +44 (0)1309 690036
e-mail: thierry@findhorn.org
url: http://www.gaia.org/findhornpress/